MASTEC

MASTECTOMY

A Patient's Guide to
Coping with Breast Surgery

by

Nancy Robinson and Ian Swash

with a Foreword by Katie Boyle

Afterword by Dr Gilbert H. Collier

THORSONS PUBLISHERS LIMITED
Wellingborough, Northamptonshire

First published March 1977
Second Impression December 1977

ISBN 0 7225 0348 2 (paperback)
ISBN 0 7225 0365 2 (hardback)

Filmset by
Specialised Offset Services Limited, Liverpool
and printed and bound in Great Britain by
Weatherby Woolnough, Sanders Road
Wellingborough, Northants

DEDICATED TO MEMBERS OF THE MASTECTOMY
ASSOCIATION OF GREAT BRITAIN

and to the many hundreds of people – professional
and lay – without whose help this book would not
have been possible.

Most of the case histories have been edited for publication,
and some of the names and localities of the volunteers
disguised.

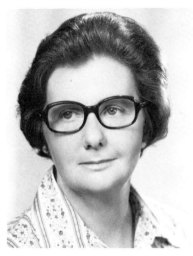

Nancy Robinson

Nancy Robinson is an Australian broadcaster and author who, in 1974, published the first definitive Australian handbook on mastectomy after-care, and in the same year founded a Mastectomy Association in that country. Coincidentally, her path crossed with that of Ian Swash who, at the same time, was setting up a Mastectomy Centre in England.

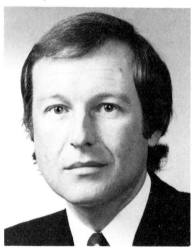

Ian Swash

Contents

List of Illustrations

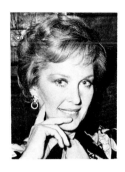

Foreword
by Katie Boyle

Up till now I still have both breasts, but all through my life I have had a 'ringside view', as it were, of breast cancer. I was just twelve years old when my stepmother, to whom I was devoted, was suddenly rushed to hospital for a mastectomy operation. Of course, at that age I didn't fully realize the nature of her illness but I'll never forget the haunting stillness and sad silence of the house when she'd left. How thrilled we were to see her back. Fragile but smiling, she became extra specially precious to us all.

That happened a long time ago but as the years have gone by mastectomies have been performed successfully on a considerable number of my friends, and most recently on my sister-in-law. What's more, in my mountainous mail at the *TV Times* I've had a steady flow of letters from women who are either facing breast surgery or want to find out how to cope with life after the experience. My heart goes out to every woman who writes to me and I've learnt a great deal about the emotional as well as the practical needs of those who have to undergo this operation.

How often I've wished I could suggest a book which would give them the answers to their questions – and to their many unwritten fears. At last I can.

Here is an entirely factual book which makes it very clear that far from being a death sentence, breast cancer is potentially one of the more curable forms of this disease, and that so far, mastectomy has proved much the best way of dealing with early cancer and saving lives. From there, it takes the patient realistically through each stage of her post-operative recovery with sound practical advice as well as deep understanding, and it's written in a friendly, conversational style which patients and their families will find easy to read. This is an honest, much needed book and I'm proud and delighted to introduce it.

KATIE BOYLE

1. Getting to Know You

This book is written primarily for the woman who has had a breast surgically removed. We hope that it will also be useful to the woman's family and to professional people involved in rehabilitation, but those are secondary considerations. Whilst we would like to think that in the next year or two women everywhere might read this or some similar book, for knowledge is both understanding and strength, our immediate aim is to help with the physical, emotional and cosmetic rehabilitation of the mastectomee.

Because the book is primarily for the new mastectomee, we'll be addressing quite a lot of what is said, directly to *you*. Of course, we can't know everyone who reads this book personally, but through contact with many hundreds of women who have had mastectomies and because we have their stories on file, we have a fair idea of a composite 'you'.

You could be quite young, maybe in your twenties and with babies or small children at home. In this case, you are probably worrying that they will fret for you, and wondering how you will cope when you go home from hospital. Or you could be in your thirties or early forties, worried that your hospitalization and convalescence will disrupt your children's studies and put extra stress on a too-busy husband.

On the other hand, you may be a young grandmother, concerned about your job or your civic responsibilities, maybe anxious as to how you can retain your image of a well-groomed matron. Or you may be sixty-plus, perhaps a widow facing this new experience without the mate who has helped you over so many hurdles in the past.

Whatever your age group, background or interests, we hope you will be able to identify with at least some of the stories and case histories that are sprinkled throughout this book. Socially, professionally and by temperament, you could come from any stratum. For all women have breasts and a woman's social standing, education and disposition make no difference when it comes to breast cancer. A few of you will have had a breast or breasts removed for reasons other than cancer. And though cancer is the most common cause of a mastectomy, the rehabilitation from the surgical removal of the breast is much the same in all cases, whether it be for cancer or for other reasons.

About the Authors

Neither of the authors is a breast amputee – indeed, one is never likely to qualify! Let's explain that statement before you close this book in disgust and say: 'Why did they give me this to read? What can these people know about if if they haven't been through it all themselves?' The simple answer stems from the fact that we care, and care enough to have spent several years (quite separately) in the research and development of a common cause. We believe that the story behind the book will convince you of our dedication, abilities and true motives, that *you* matter and that the quality of your survival matters.

Nancy Robinson is an Australian broadcaster and author who won her first literary prize at twelve and has been around the Australian press and radio scene ever since. Born at Gawler (South Australia), Nancy is only a second generation Australian on both sides, all four grandparents being English. Having married a fifth generation Australian, her two children became sixth generation Australians and are the fifth generation to live at Mannanarie, a 1200-acre farm which was taken up as virgin country by Samuel Robinson of Titchmarsh, Northamptonshire in 1872. Nancy's English forebears were a mixture of clergy, merchants and landed gentry. Reared in a series of rural rectories, the social and economic pressures of the depression and the Second World

War made a lasting impression. Her parents not only taught her to care but also to love life, a philosophy which has sustained her through recent serious illness. During the years that her own children were young, Nancy worked as a freelance on national journals, radio and local news reporting. Her first full-length book was published in 1971 and several months later she began researching and presenting her own magazine-type programme for an Adelaide radio station. Since 1971 she has had five other books published.

It was through her first commercial radio programme that Nancy became interested in mastectomy rehabilitation when she had as a guest on the programme, an Australian businesswoman who had made a remarkable adjustment to her mastectomy. At the same time, Nancy heard of another mastectomee, a woman who had virtually hidden herself away since her surgery fourteen years before. The differing reactions of these two women to an identical experience was intriguing. Nancy discovered that no library in Australia held a book suitable for the medically lay person. There were plenty of academic theses for the professionals but nothing to help a woman (or a family) suddenly confronted by mastectomy. From this point, Nancy decided to research and write a self-help book for women who had undergone the mastectomy operation, but rather than focus on the achievements of just one person, she would base her book on the experiences of many.

The fact that she was not herself a mastectomee would help. She could not be accused of being either exhibitionist or subjective in her approach. In 1974, Nancy published what has become the first definitive Australian hand-book on mastectomy aftercare, and, in the same year, she founded a Mastectomy Association in Australia.

During the period of Nancy Robinson's research into the practical and social problems of Australia's mastectomees, **Ian Swash** embarked on a venture which became no less of a crusade. At that time a manager of a British surgical company attempting to market a natural-looking breastform, he soon realized that the taboos surrounding the subject of breast cancer were so strong as to negate his company's innovation. The fact that, as a teenager, he had lost his mother to cancer personalized his interest. As Katie Boyle was later to report in a leading health magazine: 'Ian Swash found an extraordinary situation ... despite the sad fact that breast cancer is on the increase ... no one in the media would touch it ... nobody was prepared to be its first mouthpiece.' In the course of a two-year fight to create public awareness of both the problems and a partial answer, he came upon a copy of Nancy Robinson's first mastectomy book and a correspondence developed.

Over the ensuing months, numerous letters, tape recordings and manuscripts have flown to and from Australia and, happily, so has Nancy's elder daughter, Mary, who spent three months in England working at the Mastectomy Centre founded by Ian Swash. It really is the most happy coincidence that two individuals, thousands of miles apart, should choose to spend identical periods of their lives in pursuing the same philosophy, ideals and research and should finally combine their material into one book. We are grateful for the experience. Much of this book remains faithful to Nancy's original book (*Sweet Breathes the Breast*) and in this we gratefully acknowledge the co-operation of Lynton Publications, Blackwood S.A.

Help to Face the Problems

While we hope this book will help you identify with other women who have been through the same experience, and will give you many positive guides to good rehabilitation, we are not glossing over the problems. To sweep the problems under the mat, as it were – or, to use another metaphor, to sugar the pill – would be an insult to your intelligence. What we aim to do is to help you to face the problems as they arise, to conquer them one by one and to get back into the way of life just as you left it before that lump was discovered in your breast.

Ideally, you should read the book from cover to cover; but for quick reference we have added appendices and an index.

2. Betty's Story

Let us now get down to the business of helping you to adjust to life without a breast by 'meeting' the first of a number of volunteers whose stories will punctuate this book.

Betty is a petite brunette from Cumbria who has proved that with faith and determination you can turn what might first appear as a definite setback into an outright triumph.

One of the most striking things about Betty is her smile. The success of her venture into design and manufacture of mastectomy swimwear is a good reason for that smile. The origins of what has now become a most stimulating enterprise stem from her own misfortune in losing a breast together with her determination, not only to continue to live her own very full life, but also to help and encourage others to do the same. This is Betty's story:

Twelve years ago, I discovered a lump in my breast which, imagination or not, appeared to differ in size each time I re-examined it. At that time I knew nothing about mastectomy. I had, in fact, never even heard the word. Anyway, I suppose I was just as worried as if I had known the full facts. Much later I was to find that a longstanding girl-friend had undergone the operation and I just never knew. Eventually, I consulted my GP and was sent for a biopsy.

There was then a ten day gap whilst I awaited the results but as my mind was fairly occupied in coping with tonsillitis, my thoughts didn't weigh too heavily in the other direction. Then one night the surgeon from the General Hospital, where I'd had the test done, came round to see me.

Why Me?

Looking back, he was pretty wonderful really, the way he broke the news to both my husband, Bryan, and to me, but it was still an awful shock. I'm not ashamed to say that I cried a lot or that I kept asking myself why this should happen to me in particular.

Two days later I was admitted to hospital. Bryan came with me but then had to dash off to take the children, aged five and three, to their grandparents in Jarrow. I remember feeling very much alone.

The operation took place the following day and although the hospital staff were very kind to me, there wasn't the information and counselling that there is today. When I came round, I set about counselling myself simply by counting my blessings: a wonderfully understanding husband, two lovely children, a fine home and so on.

Letters, messages, cards and flowers poured in from friends near and far, some of whom I hadn't seen for ages. As they always do, these 'outward signs' helped me to feel warm again and very much part of living. Bryan is a practical, sensible man, emotionally strong in the way that a man needs to be, and although he was always there to lean upon, he had the sense never to be over-sympathetic to the point where it might detract from my own efforts to get back to normal.

On my way back from the theatre, and I'm quite sure I wasn't dreaming, the orderly had bounced my trolley into some swing doors and for a brief moment I came round before falling back into unconsciousness. For some reason, this became a common nightmare over the first few months I was home but, always with Bryan's support, I kept telling myself to appreciate what I'd got in terms of life and love as well as the material advantages that made my convalescence easier. The physiotherapist at the hospital had taught me a 'walking finger up the wall exercise' and I practised this religiously on and off throughout the day.

Shock to the Children

At our home, as in most homes with tiny children, the

bathroom door had always been open. The children and I had shared the same bathtime and the fun of bubbles and bath toys. Now I had to decide whether the shock of seeing me minus a breast might in any way alter our relationship.

Again, this is where Bryan and the surgeon came out strongly with the same good advice. Children are much more resilient than you think and far more tolerant of physical differences than adults. To suddenly shut them out of the bathroom would be more traumatic for them than just seeing an operation scar. It would create a real barrier that had never been there before and to go into contortions to keep the site of the operation away from them would affect their personalities as much as it would mine.

One thing I do feel most strongly about is that every woman should leave hospital equipped with a soft, temporary prosthesis for use until such time as she can take the weight of a permanent one. Women like me can't get by with one handkerchief; if you're well-endowed you need a few!

The Right Prosthesis

Another thing I learned from experience is that the sooner a woman gets out and about socially after she leaves hospital the better, and again the right prosthesis (temporary or permanent) can be crucial. It is essential that you are not put-off socially at a time when you should be encouraged. I remember that for the first six months when I wore one of those granulated ones (very crunchy in a cuddle!), I just wouldn't dance and when out shopping I was either consciously or unconsciously shielding myself with my arm rather than risk a tell-tale collision with another pedestrian.

Again, I owe a lot to my husband who would neither let me stay at home and mope nor settle for a second-best breast. Back I went to the hospital to find that a new fluid breastform had now become available and suddenly I felt very much the complete woman again.

Fighting Back

From there on, I really 'got up and started to fight'. Soon I was playing tennis and badminton again and swimming from the beach near my home. That's when I realized that there was a swimsuit problem for the woman who couldn't adapt her own. I'd been successful in making my own suits, evolving designs which would hold the prosthesis firmly and comfortably in place whilst swimming.

In August 1972, having completed a professional Design Course at Leicester Polytechnic, and with the sympathetic help of suppliers who were prepared to sell me small, initial quantities of materials, I launched my own mail order business in mastectomy swimwear. The success has been remarkable. Three years and four collections later, I feel as if I've been in the swimwear business all my life. Now, as we prepare the launch of yet another new range (of fashion co-ordinates), I can reflect that though life is not only swings and roundabouts, it has a very pleasant way of almost always turning out for the best.

More Secure

After my mastectomy, I tried to accept the fact that another carcinoma could develop but as the years slipped by I felt more secure. The possibility of further trouble has seemed increasingly remote and, apart for one minor flare-up, I have had every reason to be optimistic. At that time my own doctor was (as always) forthright and I was lucky to find the same attitude in both my surgeon and the consultant radiotherapist who successfully treated me. I have obviously developed a high resistance to the disease and a great deal depends on my own attitude towards the future.

I do feel it is essential for women to know as much about the problem as possible and if the re-telling of my experience helps others, then that is a very big 'something'.

Most people show at least some fear when faced with cancer and I was no exception. Though with time and good counselling at the beginning the fear does recede, it needs firmness and understanding within yourself and also within your family.

I do hope that my story may help others towards an equally successful recovery.

Though we have met a lot of mastectomees as well-adjusted as Betty and a lot of men who have been towers of strength to their wives, we chose to reproduce this story in detail because of the help-others-help-yourself business that developed as a result of Betty's mastectomy. Incidentally, we understand that as the children have grown older it has become a case of Betty and Bryan being locked out of the bathroom!

3. Preparation

Though most mastectomy surgery is now performed immediately following an initial biopsy, there are times when patients have some warning. These include cases where radiotherapy has been given some months before surgery, where 'drill biopsy' has already established the necessity for breast removal, and where a patient has had minor exploratory surgery in a local unit and pathological tests or exigencies of the hospital service have decreed that the patient should go on to some other hospital for a mastectomy.

This chapter is planned with such women in mind – though the average patient who reads this following her mastectomy will also glean some useful points from it.

You Are Not Alone

It is important for you to realize that you are far from being the first woman to face the prospect of losing a breast. Though you may not realize that you know another woman who has had this anxiety, rest assured that you *do* know at least one, probably more. So many breasts are surgically removed each week that one hospital nursing officer said: 'These days, we do more mastectomies in this place than tonsillectomies.'

You may not have realized that a particular acquaintance is a former breast patient simply because in the past such surgery was not discussed as openly as, say, the removal of tonsils. (Betty's story makes the point: 'Much later I was to find that a longstanding girl-friend had undergone the operation and I just never knew.') Anyway, if you had to list all the people you know and then to indicate whether or not they still had their tonsils, just how well do you think you would score?

Betty's initial reaction of 'Why should this happen to me?' is the most natural and understandable reaction of all. Try to calm these feelings by remembering that hundreds of thousands of other women have faced or will face the same situation. During the last decade or two, the incidence of mammary carcinoma (breast cancer) has overtaken cancer of the cervix to become the highest single site of cancer in women of the western world. (For some reason not yet clearly understood, mammary carcinoma is less prevalent in some Asiatic countries, including Japan.)

We can assure you that there will be physical, emotional and cosmetic help at hand for you during your period of recovery.

Volunteer Helpers

If you feel you would like to talk to a woman who has been through a mastectomy and has successfully adjusted to the situation, turn to Chapter 12 which is about the Mastectomy Association. This is composed entirely of volunteer helpers, each of whom has had breast surgery. If you feel you want that woman-to-woman chat *now* (as well as after the operation), phone your surgeon or family doctor to discuss it. Tell him quite frankly that you would like to have a pre-operative chat to a Mastectomy Association volunteer. He will then either contact someone on your behalf, or give you the green light to go ahead on your own.

While ill-informed friends, relatives and neighbours may have the best of intentions in relating some of the unfortunate things that happened to *their* friends, relatives or acquaintances, take what they have to say with the proverbial pinch of salt. What they relate to you just may have taken place, but it could have been a long time ago and we all know how distorted stories get in the re-telling! Remember that techniques of treatment and nursing have changed a great deal, even in recent years. One elderly woman said: 'I had my first breast off at the beginning of the war. The hospital did its best for me, but the few weeks after they took my breast off were a nightmare. Well, recently I had to have my other breast removed – that was thirty-three years since the first and I was amazed at how different everything was. The anaesthetic, the surgery itself, the dressing, the nursing – they had all improved beyond my wildest hopes.'

Remember, too, that just as every woman varies in her reaction to a mastectomy, so does every case medically. One surgeon told us: 'There are as many different types of breast cancer, as there are cells in which they occur.' Surgeons vary, too, in the techniques they employ; so please don't fall into the trap of believing that your problems will be the same ones that Mrs So-and-So had.

A Choice?

Before going on with some practical suggestions about preparing for hospital, we feel that some comment on a concern currently being touched upon in the media is necessary – namely that once cancer has been diagnosed, women are given no option as to whether or not they lose a breast.

Almost unanimously, authorities answer that, in almost every instance, they can see no justification for doing anything less than surgical removal of the breast. Most feel strongly that a woman has neither the specialized knowledge nor the objectivity to make the decision for herself.

From the other side of the coin, we would say that we have found only a handful of women who would have *wanted* to have a say in the matter, despite the protestations of a few vocal militants to the contrary. Most patients are prepared to submit to what their medical team considers the best procedure; but if at this time you are having serious doubts, if you are one of that minority who considers that the patient is manipulated like a puppet on a string, then *do* something about it *now*. Don't wait until after surgery and then carry a chip on your shoulder for ever and a day.

If you and your husband want to discuss the facts further, ring your surgeon to ask if you may visit him together. At the same time, your family doctor should also be a great help. Put your cards on the table. 'We wonder if a mastectomy is really necessary. May we have a simple explanation, a round table conference about it?' If the explanations of surgeon and/or GP still don't satisfy you, then ask for another opinion.

It *is* your body; you *do* have a right to know what is being done to it and why. On the other hand, you must trust your medical team, and realize that you are not really equipped to make the necessary decisions. And as you are probably not quite yourself emotionally at present (after all, it isn't every day that a woman is told that she has cancer and must have a breast removed), do try to take some rational member of the family along with you to any appointment you may have to discuss the pros and cons of the case. So many medical people have told us they feel much of what they say to the patient, either before surgery or shortly afterwards, falls on deaf ears. You have had a shock, so do not rely only upon your reaction or memory of what the surgeon tells you. We applaud those surgeons who make a point of calling the husband in for a chat, explaining what will be done, why it will be done and the patient's possible reactions. So don't get uptight if your husband has a call from the surgeon or from your family physician. They are having a sensible, man-to-man talk, just as you may wish to have a woman-to-woman talk with someone who knows what this is all about.

Time to Think

Most surgeons, when arranging to remove a lump for a microscopic examination, explain to the patient that if it proves to be malignant, they will go straight ahead with the removal of the breast and any surrounding tissues they think necessary. Only a minority say: 'No, I'd like time to prepare, to think. Give me a few days in between, please.' If you fall into that category, do not be afraid to ask or even to demand. The surgeon may advise against any delay or a second anaesthetic but, on the other hand, he may be quite agreeable to giving you a few days in which to make preparations for the mastectomy if it means you are going to be happier about it.

Preparing for Hospital

No two hospitals are exactly alike, any more than any two women about to have mastectomies are alike. But most of you will have had some experience of general hospital routine.

Most hospitals issue a list, but if unsure of what you are allowed to take into hospital with you, either phone the hospital and ask for the relevant ward sister or the Admissions Department, or just use your common sense. Err on the side of taking too little rather than too much, because storage space is at a premium in many present-day hospitals, and your family can bring you additional comforts as you need them.

On the other hand, a patient travelling from an out-lying area may feel more self-sufficient by having a few additional personal belongings with her. Most hospitals have baggage rooms where empty cases can go after being unpacked. By negotiating with the staff, you can often arrange to have an extra case with spare odds and ends in it, likewise deposited in the baggage room. This can give a sense of security to the country patient away from her home surroundings.

Some older women, rather than worry anyone to do their washing, have spent most of their post-mastectomy stay in hospital clad in hospital gowns. This idea will not, of course, appeal to the woman wanting to pretty herself, but we mention it simply to reassure you that if you do run short of your own nighties or pyjamas, then there is always hospital linen available to fill the gap. You would be surprised to know what even small hospitals have stowed away in their Goodie Bags, ready for any emergencies.

If you know you are going to have private facilities, you may like to pack a little jar with soap powder so you can rinse out your nighties and briefs and hang them to dry – that is, after you are getting about, which you should be quite quickly. If organized drying facilities are not available, the chances are that you will still find somewhere to hang your clothes overnight – maybe near or even on the central heating unit. Do take a few wire coat-hangers with you, for as any seasoned traveller or hospital patient will tell you, there is nothing you can't hang on, around, or over a wire hanger if you have enough ingenuity. The old-time, starchy matrons who expected hospitals to look as sterile and de-humanized as they smelt are becoming a thing of the past; nursing officers are human and most realize that women get well more quickly if they feel independent – and rinsing out your clothes is part of that necessary independence.

Telephone

A telephone can be a great comfort, both to patient and family. Private patients often have the use of a bedside telephone, although provision of this facility varies from hospital to hospital. If you feel that a telephone is an essential part of your private care, enquire about it as soon as you know the date of your admission.

However, there are also public telephones around every hospital, where walking patients can ring out. If you can't see where such phones are located, ask a member of the hospital staff to direct you. Like most public phone boxes anywhere, hospital ones are often minus a directory – so take with you a diary or notebook in which you have written the numbers of people you may want to contact.

What to Take

When packing your hospital requirements, include a few tiny safety-pins, a needle, some thread, some of your husband's large white handkerchiefs, and a pure silk scarf if you have one. This kit is to help you experiment with a temporary breastform so that you leave the hospital feeling at least partially 'compensated'. More and more hospitals now hold stocks of a specially made, ultra-light post-operative breastform suitable for wear during the first six to eight weeks after the operation, until the chest tissue settles down and is able to accept a specially weighted, permanent breastform. However, unless you are absolutely certain that your hospital is one of the enlightened ones, we would advise you to pack the items listed above.

Also remember to pack some postage stamps, writing paper and envelopes and some small change for newspapers and telephone – as well as the more obvious toilet requisites. And for reasons we shall see later, take something small to crochet or knit.

It is important for you to know that as far as actual surgery and nursing treatment is concerned, the National Health patient is no less privileged than the fee-paying patient. Many patients, whatever their circumstances, prefer the comradeship of a public ward to privacy at any price. It depends to a great extent on your attitudes and personality. Some mastectomees who have gone into hospital as private patients later wish they had opted for the post-operative companionship of others as well as a saving of money.

Life in hospital is the same as life outside. It's what you make it, except that the philosophy is telescoped into a smaller world for the time you are there.

Knowledge of Cosmetic Aids

Don't worry if this is as far as you have time to read before leaving for hospital. Take the book with you, and when you feel well enough you can continue with it. In the meantime, if there is any particular aspect of your recovery that you are wondering about, we suggest you refer to the index at the back of the book.

If you have time, do skim through the chapters on prostheses. Some women are helped by investigating in person the cosmetic aids that will be available to them after their surgery. For instance, a thirty-year-old woman who knew she was to have both breasts removed said that her doctor had given her the address of a skilled and discreet corsetiere. 'I made time to go and have a look at what was available,' she said, 'and was thus reassured that to all outward appearances I would be normal. This knowledge helped my acceptance of surgery and in turn that helped my rehabilitation.'

4. Dented But Not Daunted

It is not for us, or any other lay-person for that matter, to offer you a prognosis (i.e. a prediction of your future, medically). Only your surgeon and/or your family doctor can speak to you about such matters. Try not to pester nursing staff about this. Nurses can be a valuable link in your chain of rehabilitation, but it is not fair to question them about your long-term chance of survival.

You have probably heard of women who have died of breast cancer. Yes, some do die; but in this book you will meet (as we have met) others who have lived useful and happy lives for five, ten, twenty, thirty and more years after having a mastectomy.

'The Dread Disease'

It is only natural that you are apprehensive about your future. Cancer has been a 'dirty' word in our society, ingrained into our culture amidst a host of legends, hushed whispers, hoodoos, fears and half-truths. You may be of the generation that would not even use the word cancer, referring to it only as 'the dread disease'. All your adult life you have hoped that cancer would never catch up with *you*. And now that it has, you may be finding it very hard to accept. It is important for all of us to get cancer into perspective.

George Crile Jnr, MD, in his book *Cancer and Commonsense* (published by Robert Hale, London), tells the story of a 75-year-old woman, paralysed and unable to speak, being brought to hospital in an ambulance. She had been referred by her family doctor with a lump in the thyroid gland. The GP thought that her paralysis might be the result of a cancer of the thyroid that had spread to the brain. If so, he hoped that radio-active iodine could be used to destroy the cancer and give the patient a chance of recovery.

X-rays were taken and trace tests with radio-active iodine. The family, a son and two daughters, called each day to inquire about their mother. The old lady paralysed and stuporous in bed. At last the tests were completed. There was no evidence of cancer. 'There is nothing that can be done,' the family were told. 'Your mother has suffered a stroke from a broken blood vessel; the brain is irreparably damaged. There is no operation or treatment that can help.' The eldest daughter leaned forward, tense and with a quaver in her voice, asked: 'Did you find cancer?' 'There was no cancer,' I replied. 'Thank God!' the family exclaimed.

What a strange attitude! Had cancer been present it might have been permanently cured. *Nothing* could be done about the haemorrhage in the brain. The family were concerned not so much with the possibility of curing their mother as with a blind instinctive dread of a word. It was not cancer itself that the family feared, it was the word 'cancer' and its connotations of fear.

In some communities, the legends and half-truths surrounding cancer have proved much harder to destroy than cancer itself.

Facing Up to It

In talking with many well-adjusted people who know they have had cancerous growths removed, the words 'face it' have occurred over and over again. On the other hand, the patient who tries to hide from the fact, who pretends to herself that it was not really cancer, finds rehabilitation very difficult.

Women who resign themselves to the fact of having malignant tissue removed from their bodies and who have faith and hope for the future, can be at peace with themselves and their families.

Kate's Story

Kate from Cardiff is an attractive auburn-haired woman who

looks a good ten years younger than her forty-seven years. Her story illustrates the importance of attitudes.

I first noticed a tiny indentation above my right breast. I felt around the area and it seemed to be a bit thick. Next day I went to my doctor. He said that I should have it examined at the hospital.

I went to the out-patients, where I was examined by a consultant. He said that I had a lump that should be removed and arranged for me to be admitted. I felt sheer panic at the thought of going to hospital when I wasn't even ill.

After a week of tests, I was told that my right breast would have to be removed and a biopsy would be taken on the left side. If there was doubt, the left breast would also be removed. Very gently the consultant broke the news to me. He also telephoned my husband. My husband was a wonderful strength. When we talked I felt that we were fighting the same fight and in squaring up to it we had become even closer. Before this, I had felt relief; at least I knew what I had to face.

During the week of tests, I hadn't known what was happening or what was wrong with me. Knowing, I felt a growing sense of calm. I put all my trust in the doctors and having accomplished that, I didn't really worry any more. The companionship of patients in the ward was a blessing. They were sympathetic but tried to make me think 'positive'. After I'd had the surgery, for removal of both breasts, I really made up my mind to get well quickly by doing the simple things.

For example, I decided to eat everything brought to me at mealtimes in order to get my strength back fast. Again, I like to keep my hair looking nice and anticipated great difficulty curling and combing. Anyway, I got my husband to bring my heated rollers in to me and using them twice a day helped with the arm excercises and very soon I was curling other patients hair in the ward and keeping myself busy.

Four days after my operation, I was told everything was fine and there would be no further treatment needed. It was the most marvellous thing to be told. A young nurse asked me if she could do my case history for her exams. She said she was a sucker for a happy ending! That was six years ago. I'm truly very well – in fact, I feel better than I used to feel years ago. I have much more energy and enthusiasm for life and rarely feel tired. So many good things have happened to me since that operation. My three children are grown up now but six years ago when I was facing what I first thought of as disaster, they were only twelve, fourteen and fifteen.

My husband and I are celebrating our silver wedding next year. I am feeling so well and happy now that I look forward to our golden wedding together.

Overcoming the Fear

During your convalescence, you may like to read a book that develops these points further. *Determined to Live*, written by the Rev. Brian Hession and published by Peter Davies, London, is the story of one man's triumph over the fear of cancer. You could gain much strength and comfort from this book even if you are not a practising Christian.

Do try to get on top of fear; for fear is exhausting.

Hope, on the other hand, is exhilarating.

Brian Hession wrote: 'Hope is the most precious possession any of us can have. Coupled with courage it can work wonders ... While there is hope, there is life enough for the next day and that day may be the turning point.'

For the woman who has had a malignant breast removed, there is a double amount of facing and accepting to be done. She must face not only the fact of cancer, but also what she feels to be a glaring disfigurement.

Actually, with the help of a good surgical fitter and a well-informed dress adviser, the 'disfigurement' is not obvious to other people. But we do know how you feel about this at present, and once again assure you that plenty of help is now available. Our hearts go out to the many women who in the past were given no guidance at all on where to go for cosmetic help. Many went for years and years without a prosthesis, or proper swimwear or the knowledge of how to adapt their clothes so that their breastlessness would not be apparent. We have spoken with scores of them; but the barriers of poor communication and professional myopia have tumbled rapidly during the past year or so and we think that the day of the uninformed mastectomee will soon be past.

A Feeling of Lost Femininity

The aspect you may be finding the most difficult to face is feeling that part of your femininity has gone. Lots of women have told us that they felt 'only half a woman' after their mastectomy, and that it took them a long time to adjust to what they refer to as 'being made neuter'. Of course, all that is poppycock, really. You have not lost your femininity at all. Surely, your womanhood rests on much more than your mammary glands. Right now it could be difficult for you to believe otherwise but let us assure you that well-adjusted mastectomees in time feel no loss of femininity; and that their husbands can adapt their love-making, too. It isn't always easy for them, but with help they can do it.

Over the centuries, man's worship of the female body has taken many forms.

Historically, there have been times when breasts were idolized more than they are now, and times when ample bustlines were considered so vulgar that girls bound their developing breasts with linen and even plates of iron.

You have lost your breast in an age when, by and large, society overdoes the importance of it, so in learning to face the situation, don't worry if you sometimes feel rather bitchy towards women with two whole breasts, or if seeing bra commercials on television or splashed across the Press upsets you for a while. This is quite a common early reaction.

On the other hand, we could name several hundred women popularly regarded as sex-symbols whose attraction depends on their overall appearance and general 'sexuality' rather than on one specific area of their anatomy.

'Whatever anyone may suggest to the contrary, I'm happy to report that a love affair still begins at eye level and achieves its satisfaction well south of the bust. That was something I was glad about *before* the operation and I have no reason to change my attitude,' said one sensible young single woman whose name we must omit!

A Challenge

You may also be interested to know about another friend of

ours, a model who, unknown to almost everyone, underwent a simple mastectomy some six or seven years ago. When she was recently asked to model a foundation her first reaction was to turn the job down. Her second was to accept it as a challenge and her delight was in coming through the session completely undetected! Such is the degree of sophistication of one of the latest breastforms.

Judging by what other women have told us, you will in time get over any resentment towards the naturally full-busted woman. That phrase 'in time' seems to be the key. An athlete does not win Olympic gold medals the first time he competes in a club contest. It may sound trite and jingoistic, but do remember that if you keep climbing step by step, you will reach the top of the staircase – in time. The strength of Kate's philosophy is in its simplicity. 'I really made up my mind to get well quickly by doing the simple things.'

Setting Yourself Goals to Reach

One of the many women who wrote to Nancy Robinson said: 'A few days after my mastectomy, I decided I would give myself goals to reach. I had one big, long-distance goal. Our daughter was being married overseas, exactly three months after the day of my surgery. I determined to be well enough, adjusted enough and well-groomed enough to get to the wedding with my husband, and to have my family proud of me. Each day I would think of some new but often quite trivial goal to strive for, and then I would add it to a list. Almost every day I was able to cross of something on my "little goal" list but it might not have been the thing I had written down the day before. It still gave me so much satisfaction to know I was reaching those minor goals on the way to achieving my major goal. That was three years ago now. I did get to our daughter's wedding, they were proud of me and now we're expecting our daughter and her baby girl to arrive home next week.'

Elizabeth, a country woman who had a breast removed when she was thirty-two, told how she had persuaded the surgeon to let her leave hospital a day earlier than scheduled.

'I got home on the Thursday,' she said, 'and took over at a final rehearsal with my choir on the Saturday afternoon. On the Sunday night I conducted them through "The Messiah" and sang a solo. I'm sure feeling so responsible for that performance forced me into regaining my confidence sooner than would have been possible otherwise. The gift of life is far too wonderful to waste it in self-pity.'

A voluntary helper wrote: 'Do assure your friend that her present miseries are only a temporary phase and that in a few months' time she will feel enormously better. If she would like to phone me any evening just to talk things over I would be delighted to hear from her. It seems strange to me now that I was so embarrassed about my condition this time last year. I shall be spending Christmas at Ambleside once again, and I am looking forward very much to roaming over the fells during the day and dancing most of the night.'

Accepting and Adjusting

Yet another woman told us: 'A friend who had her breast off about a year before I had my mastectomy came to see me in hospital one afternoon. She's a bit of a rough diamond on the outside, this friend of mine, but underneath all that, she's as soft as a kitten. Well, I told her I didn't know quite how I was going to face a new life. She laughed and took hold of my hand. "Look here, silly. It isn't a *new* life. What you're facing, Jen, is just the continuation of the old life, only you're a bit dented, that's all. I know you well enough to know you can adjust. It's a continuation, Jen, that's all. Maybe a new chapter, but definitely not a bloody new book. Of course you wouldn't want to leave behind all your old life and start a new one. It's too damned good, isn't it?" I found her rough philosophy very helpful and that night, when my husband visited me, I told him: "I might be dented but I'm not daunted." My family made quite a joke of that for months afterwards.'

Janet is fifty-six and had a breast removed in 1968. The special circumstances of Janet's case allowed for a two-week waiting period between the tests and the operation itself.

I remember, very clearly, the initial shock of being told that I had cancer but I do feel that the waiting period that followed the tests was helpful in my case. It allowed me to come to terms with myself and my condition and the importance of life itself.

During this period, I astounded myself by making the conscious decision not to tell my family either about the cancer or losing a breast until it was all over. Although my husband and four very grown-up sons were just as strong and just as sensible as they are today, there seemed no real point in making them unhappy for me or in saying or doing anything that might alter the normal atmosphere of our home. Perhaps in a way, I was testing my own strength. With hindsight, I believe that I made the right decision *for me*, but that is not to say it would be the right decision for others.

In the event, my husband only learned about the mastectomy when it had taken place and I was looking well, up and about. If anything, my attitude increased his regard for me and I felt that having come through this battle unaided, there was little or nothing that I couldn't overcome in the future. My husband then broke the news to the rest of the family.

Later, when I underwent radiotherapy treatment – twelve sessions, two per week – I gained additional strength and encouragement from both my family and the kindly staff of the radiotherapy department. I'd been told that the treatment might be unpleasant but throughout I held on to the conviction that I was *winning* over cancer. Light meals, rest at the proper time, and at no time was I sick!

The whole point of my story is that I had not been known for my bravery! But once I got over the initial shock of what was to happen, I accepted that mastectomy operation and subsequent radiotherapy as my only possible life-saver. As the treatment was something that I couldn't live without, I decided I must try to welcome the chance it afforded rather than just bemoan the loss of a breast. That way, although the experience wasn't pleasant and no one would volunteer for it, it didn't feel like pointless suffering and, let's face it, I was just as much alive as I'd always been.

After the operation, I made the point of being as open about it as I possibly could. In talking to other women, I find that many anticipate totally the wrong reaction from their menfolk. They think that husband, boyfriend, family will be put off, whereas I'm convinced that if the relationships were sound to start with, it's highly unlikely that breast removal will make any difference.

Perhaps I'm luckier than some, but I don't think I'm any luckier than Mrs Average. There are some wonderful families about. I have a super husband and four very level-headed sons who share a strong sense of perspective and a strong sense of fun. When I was young, I used to fly old bi-planes and the family joke is that from bi-planes I then went on to invent the mono-bosom! In the same vein, if, in the early days, I stretched up and my falsie slipped, I'd be accused of flying 'one wing low'. In fact, a murmured 'one wing low, mum' was a useful code in 1968 when, in the main, prostheses and specialist bra-lines were not quite so sophisticated as they are today! Again, it was a problem easily conquered with a pantie-corselet – but how could I ever be embarrassed *outside* the family with that sort of conditioning *inside*!

Nowadays, I have a whole wardrobe of entirely feminine mastectomy apparel and no cosmetic problems. Quite honestly, I'd defy anyone to ever detect *you* have had a mastectomy unless you choose to tell them.

I must confess I thought twice about mentioning my 'go-it-alone' attitude towards the operation itself, but again mastectomy operations aren't restricted to married women. Some patients are single or far from home, and so to a certain extent are 'going it alone' anyway. Whatever one's personal circumstances, a complete recovery *is* possible, winning is enjoyable and living continues to be such tremendous fun.

A Sense of Humour

What a wonderful attitude and how good it was that, like Janet, so many of the women who helped in our research had a sense of humour. With life in general, but in this situation in particular, a sense of humour is a priceless asset.

For instance, there was the mastectomee who, with a twinkle in her lovely eyes, referred to herself as 'one lamp Lulu'; there was another who referred to her prosthesis as 'Martha the second'; and another who told hilarious tales of how, on an organized bus trip, she kept her money in her 'treasure chest' by removing the teased wool stuffing from her 'soft' breastform. Likewise, there was the Australian traveller who took out her prosthesis when approaching a state-border fruit block to replace it with several contraband mandarin oranges she wanted to eat as she drove.

Many stories, told against themselves by mastectomees, testify to the degree of readjustment that has been made. It should be stated that most of these stories emanate from the days before the present ranges of highly sophisticated breastforms became available. One 'hen-party' piece is the story of how a very beautiful woman had filled a balloon with water and gone to a dance. Unfortunately, the balloon burst and she soaked her partner's suit! Another woman, a bilateral, decided it was 'high-time' she invested in a new swimsuit when she found her two prostheses gently floating away from her across the swimming bath. As this gifted raconteur was heard to remark later: 'Time and tide wait for no one!'

Stories from women who have left their homes without remembering to insert their prostheses are legion. Again, these mastectomees tell the stories against themselves with a great deal of honest mirth, yet we realize this degree of readjustment has come only after a considerable passage of time. Not that a sense of humour cannot rear its soul-healing head at any time, mind you. There was the husband who, on leaving his wife at the hospital ready for a mastectomy the following morning, said: 'Well, old girl, keep your chin up.' And her classic reply: 'Actually it isn't my chin that's the trouble.'

Mary, who had worn two hearing aids since childhood, said after both breasts were removed: 'All I need now is a wooden leg or two and I'm sure my husband would qualify for the man whose wife has the most spare parts. But he still loves me. He doesn't find me repulsive. In fact, he's always telling me how nice I look and we can joke about all my spare parts.'

Another family, with older teenage children, have built a topical, private joke around 'mum' as the sequel to television's 'Six Million Dollar Man'. Since a recent Italian holiday when mum got her bottom pinched, she has described herself as 'sexier and with higher viewing figures!'

We could go on and on telling you amusing, *human* tit-bits, of how women have faced their loss of a breast with good cheer; but we have no doubt that you and your family will collect your own little portfolio of such stories.

5. The Build Up: Commercial Prostheses

There are a number of ways a surgeon can perform a mastectomy, and no two mastectomees will look *exactly* alike. Just as no two paintings are completely identical, and a connoisseur will be able to define the work – so it is with mastectomies. Indeed, a highly skilled mastectomy fitter who has worked with the same District Hospital for a number of years may instinctively recognize the work of a particular surgeon. On a national basis, there are many surgeons and a great many mastectomy patients. Suffice it to say, then, that mastectomies fall into three categories:

1, *Partial* – where part of the breast is removed.
2. *Simple* – where only the breast (or part of the breast) is removed.
3. *Radical* – where much more tissue (muscles, glands, lymph nodes etc.) is taken away to make sure that all the malignant cells are removed.

Choose a Good Fitter
Naturally, radical surgery makes the restoration of your figure to its former shape a more complicated job for the professional fitter or corsetiere. More complicated, more challenging but *far from impossible*. This is where the skill, care and understanding of the dedicated fitter comes into the picture. The slipshod fitter, on the other hand, will sell you a prosthesis and that's that. She will do nothing to help you fill in the hollows left between breast and neck, for instance, or the hollows left under the arm. Without such 'wings' or

extension pieces built on to your prosthesis, close-fitting clothes will never hang quite properly. At the other extreme, the dedicated fitter-corsetiere is fully trained on a continuing basis by a major manufacturer or distributor of breastforms. This means that she will be familiar with all the different types of prostheses currently available. Our experience of the very best fitters is that they will recommend only the prosthesis that is right for *you*, without bias towards any particular manufacturer. Remember what we said at the start of this chapter – no two mastectomees are exactly the same, no two operations are the same in the minutest detail – and therefore the prosthesis that is right for your neighbour may not be the one that is exactly right for you. Insist on seeing all that *are* available, but in the final analysis be guided by a good fitter. Like everything else, you will be quick to recognize a good one when you see her.

National Health Supplies

You are legally entitled to a prosthesis on hospital prescription, under the National Health Scheme (and, morally, a proper fitting service) but the interpretation of this entitlement varies from hospital to hospital. Some hospitals fail to stock or obtain items from the full range of prostheses available to them under manufacturers' contracts with the Department of Health. We think this is unfortunate.

However, there is every reason to believe than an accumulation of individual complaints from the more outspoken, together with the sensitive and diplomatic approaches of the Mastectomy Association on behalf of the silent majority, will ultimately ensure that *all* hospitals stock the full range of prostheses accepted under contract by the Department of Health.

We are tempted to say that a concerted public outcry would not come amiss in cases where hospitals do not order the full range of breastforms available for NHS prescription. But what you may not be able to obtain under the NHS initially is always available privately, and the number of recalcitrant hospitals seems to be decreasing despite 'budgetary problems'. We appreciate that budgetary problems *do* exist, that hospital funds must serve many demands; and yet our several years' research in the mastectomy field has served merely to reinforce our belief that, come what may, the full range of breastforms and a proper fitting service should be made available to every hospital patient. A national increase in the prescription charge for the more sophisticated products would be preferable to non-availability in certain areas. However, this is another instance where there is nothing to prevent you, the patient, making enquiries *before* your admission. *For* you *matter; and the quality of your survival matters.*

Breastforms

There are six main brands of prosthesis available in Britain today.

The Poisette. This range of external prostheses offers varying sizes and styles which do look, feel and move like a natural breast and are virtually undetectable under normal clothing or even swimwear. They are composed of a smooth, flesh-coloured silicone skin filled with a soft mobile silicone gel which closely resembles breast tissue and has virtually the same specific gravity. The unique qualities of these silicone prostheses means that they can be placed against the chest without any special covering and can be used with the patient's normal brassiere, thus presenting a life-like contour, matching the normal breast in weight, texture, temperature and mobility.

The Poisette quickly assumes body temperature and, being non-absorbent to fluids etc., will not assimilate body odours. Ordinary toilet soap and water is sufficient to keep it clean. It can be dried with a towel ready for use again.

Because of the silicone composition, these prostheses will withstand extremes of temperature and should they be pierced with pins etc., will not leak or lose shape – only lacerations will cause irreparable damage. Important points are that no special brassiere is required and the prosthesis will last for many years without deterioration.

Promotion of the Poisette is mainly directed at the private

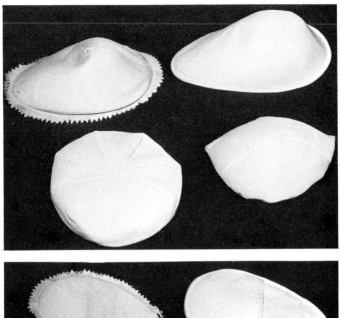

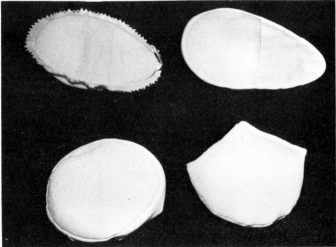

2. Four types of prostheses (breastforms) commonly used in Britain. Top picture shows fronts and bottom picture shows backs of same four prostheses.

Top-left: Tru-life *(fluid)*; *Top right:* Confidante *(fluid/air) Bottom left:* Malpro *(granules)*; *Bottom right:* Spenfil *(temporary prosthesis for immediate post-operative wear.)*

market, but there are certain circumstances in which it can be prescribed. The problem then becomes one of cost, and for each prescription, the hospital concerned is involved in submitting what is known as a 'special (i.e. individual) estimate' for approval by the Department of Health.

Although the vast majority of women who obtain this breastform do so privately, many have said that the overall benefits far outweigh the purchase price.

The Confidante. This is the only prosthesis cleverly combining both fluid and air. A fluid centre contains a non-toxic gel to give natural breast weight and balance, and an outer skin provides a medium whereby only the slightest addition of air maintains natural fluctuation of breast contour. The air is inserted by means of a straw and self-sealing valve.

The prosthesis mirrors the appearance, texture and feel of the true breast and is impervious to chlorinated pool or sea-water. The size range goes from a 32-inch to a 46-inch bust and from approximately $3\frac{3}{4}$ ounces to 26 ounces in weight. The prosthesis comes complete with its own cover of soft,

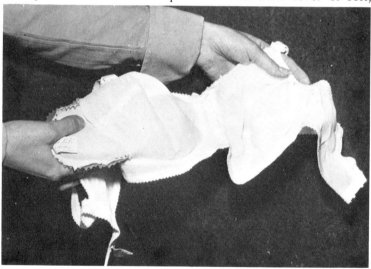

3. A *Tru-life* prosthesis being fitted into the pocket of a mastectomy bra.

white or flesh-coloured material and slips snugly into the pocket of a mastectomy bra. Ordinary toilet soap and water is sufficient to keep it clean but great care must be taken to avoid damage such as pin-pricks. In other words, treat it as gently as you would your real breast. The Confidante can be obtained via the NHS, but you may not get it automatically and may even have to order it privately in certain areas. It will last from one to four years.

The Tru-Life. This is a fluid-filled artificial breast with a thin layer of foam-back and a removable covering of synthetic fabric. Like the Confidante, it has good, fluid mobility, a wide size-range and fits into a pocket built into your bra. Flesh coloured with a natural-looking nipple, it is really quite life-like. Again, care should be taken to avoid pin-pricks etc., but under normal conditions, this breastform will last from one to four years.

The Malpro. This prosthesis contains a mixture of ceramic granules and foam particles for weight and movement, and has a washable outside cover. Like Confidante and Tru-Life, it is intended for wear with a specially adapted bra. It is the least expensive of the four main brands. (Both Malpro and Tru-Life are widely available under the NHS.)

Carefree. This prosthesis is similar in construction to the Poisette (i.e. it is a silicone gel encased in a flesh-coloured silicone skin) but is more natural in appearance. The product, which has a remarkably natural feel, moulds itself to the chest wall so closely that any irregularities are taken up quite painlessly. The fact that it is completely seamfree makes for greater durability and ease of fitting. The manufacturers claim that there is no skin reaction – so keeping the prosthesis odourless.[1]

The Spenco. A silicone breastform that comes in two shapes, ten sizes in each shape, and in beige and brown skin tones.

The *Tear Drop* shape is recommended for the woman who has had a radical mastectomy, while the *Heart Shape* form is designed for the woman who has had a simple mastectomy. At

[1]We understand that Patientcare are soon to introduce a second, more sophisticated prosthesis under the name *Breastforme*.

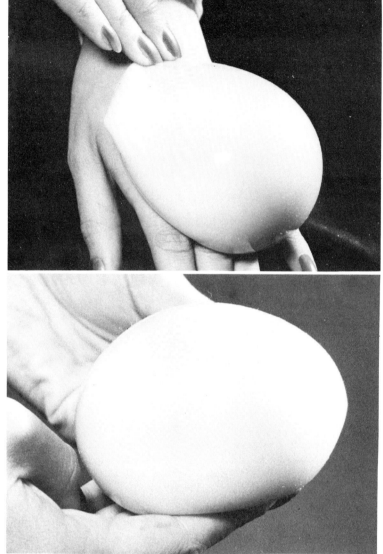

Photos courtesy of Patientcare Mastectomy Centres (Ross & Hilliard)

4. Pictures show the lifelike properties of the silicone breastform.

the present time the Spenco prosthesis is probably the least expensive of the silicone forms.

We have said that not every hospital stocks every type of prosthesis, and neither does every private surgical fitter. The addresses of the UK distributors for all these breastforms are shown in the appendix. Literature is available, and you may like to write to the distributors for brochures and the names of your nearest suppliers – that is, trained corsetieres who would fit you. In these circumstances, it would help if you were to indicate your nearest town or city and include a medium-sized stamped, addressed envelope. These fitter-corsetieres work from home and arrangements can be made for you to meet with the fitter either at her home or yours.

Shop Around

Unfortunately, Britain lags way behind other countries (the USA, in particular) in accepting mastectomy apparel as retail merchandise. To date only a very small percentage of stores and corsetry shops provide anything like a proper service. Having said that, you may just be lucky enough to find someone in your own home town. So ask around, by all means, but don't rush to the conclusion that the large stores are necessarily the best places; our experience is that, mostly, they couldn't care a fig.

Arguably, there is no other area of merchandise that can be so completely marketed to stores, with free training programmes, publicity and sales help and a real opportunity to gratify customers and win their unshakeable loyalty to the store for both mastectomy and other purchases. In the face of this, the arguments of some stores' buyers – 'too little profit', 'too difficult', and so on – appear to be both morally bad and commercially nonsensical.

Installing a basic range of mastectomy apparel either in a specialist corsetry shop or department store is not going to cost a lot. Obviously, mastectomy-wear turns over in a different way from other body fashions but one would think that low stock-levels and frequent re-ordering would be infinitely preferable to some of those massive bulk purchases which hang around all year and eventually are marked down to be 'moved out' in a Sale.

Faced with this innate resistance from stores' buyers, two major distributors have now established their own centres in London's West End, and television personality Katie Boyle, whose own stepmother had a mastectomy, has gone on record as saying that she will not rest until there is a Mastectomy Centre in the lingerie department of every major store. Knowing Katie for the determined person she is, we have every reason to assume that, in time, she will be successful.

As far as hospitals go, we feel that the various types of breast prostheses should be displayed in a small fitting room or cubicle and that the patient should have time to conduct her own examination either alone, or with her husband or a friend and, if she wishes, seek further information from the Appliance Officer. It is important that she is free to make up her own mind which types would suit her and would be most acceptable.

Manufacturers and Distributors

Meanwhile, until those responsible get themselves sorted out, do not hesitate to contact manufacturers and distributors direct or to make those subtle enquiries *before* your admission to hospital. Remember, for your peace of mind, that the dedicated surgical fitter can *always* be found as a result of your own enquiries and that a list of key addresses, including that of the Mastectomy Association, is contained in the appendices of this book.

In some areas you may find a local supplier of prostheses listed in the yellow pages of your telephone directory 'disguised' under the headings 'Foundation Garment Consultants' or 'Surgical Appliance Manufacturers and Suppliers'. And some senior members of nursing staff are well-equipped to give you information about the local scene, as are some radiotherapists and their staffs.

By one method or another, then, or by a combination of all these means, you should be able to put together the complete 'how and where' of what breastforms are available.

If all else fails, write to us, care of the publishers, and we will give you all the help we can – but please enclose a stamped, addressed envelope for our reply. Obviously, with no commercial backing, and with other projects to consider, we cannot commit ourselves to a heavy mail load, but we make the offer in the hope that no mastectomee need have her full rehabilitation jeopardized through lack of local information. The message is, then, 'if you need us, call us'.

Better Communication

All things considered, you are relatively lucky. You have had your mastectomy in an era when, at last, the subject is being publicly aired. In fact, the climate of feeling has changed so dramatically since we began our research that there is even a chance of people becoming tired of hearing about breast removal and its aftermath. At least, because of this swing to better communication, you will know where to go for help, rather than having to wait twenty years for the information! And you will know that others will share your experience.

In addition to the cosmetic value of a prosthesis, there is the very important fact of the weight of a well-fitting one giving you physical balance. This is, of course, particularly so with big-busted women, but is also evident in some quite petite mastectomees. If not adequately weighted on the side of the mastectomy, a woman may become clumsy. She may even trip and fall frequently, or lose her balance on kitchen ladders, or hunch a shoulder or twist her spine to 'compensate'. As you can imagine, all these bring their own problems and, prevention being better than cure, this is where a properly balanced prosthesis can act in a preventive way.

Prices

With inflationary trends, we hesitate to quote prices in this book, yet not to do so would be to deprive some of you of essential information. We therefore qualify the following figures by stressing that these prices are meant to serve only as a rough guide based on information available to us at the time of writing. At present all hospitals provide, on prescription, a free initial issue of two prostheses for the bilateral mastectomee and one prosthesis for the single mastectomee. Some hospitals will also allow a basic bra as a separate prescription item on payment of a fee of £2, or arrange for you to make a low-cost purchase through a visiting supplier. The more enlightened hospitals will, in addition to these items, supply a soft 'temporary' prosthesis (suitable for short-term post-operative wear) either free or on payment of a small charge.

We are sorry that we have to go on saying 'some hospitals will do this' or 'some hospitals will do that' but until such time as the Health Service decides to 'get-it-together' and realizes the importance of doing so, we must continue to point out the differences. These differences are not simply regional: what you get and the service you get can vary considerably from one side of the town to the other.

Prices for the *private* supply and fitting of a prosthesis vary only slightly. At the time of going to print, a rough guide would be: granular, up to £6; fluid or fluid-air, up to £18; silicone (which has an indefinite life), between £31 and £51 according to type and size.

The First Fitting

When is a patient ready for her first prosthesis? This varies, just as every other facet of rehabilitation varies from woman to woman. Scar tissue takes longer to heal in some women than in others, while others have fluid problems for many weeks after surgery. And some women are emotionally ready for a prosthesis-fitting much sooner than others. Radiotherapy, too, can delay the time when you can wear a proper breastform, if for no other reason than the practical one of having dye marks on the skin, which could injure the fabric of an expensive prosthesis.

Temporary Prostheses

The soft 'temporary' prosthesis has been designed for you to wear during the first few weeks following your mastectomy. It will help to restore your natural figure, yet exerts no pressure on the area of the incision while complete healing (both external and internal) is taking place. Later, when you are quite accustomed to wearing a weighted, permanent prosthesis throughout the day, you will find that a soft prosthesis can still have its uses from time to time, either as bedtime wear or as a travelling 'reserve'. There are three types of lightweight prostheses available in the commercial field, each costing less than £2. However, don't rush into buying one until you have made absolutely certain that your own hospital is not a supplier. Despite variations in content, in effect these prostheses are very much the same:

1. **Spenfil.** This lightweight breastform is made from fibrefil, filled with Kodel, and is available in five sizes; extra small, small, medium, large and extra large.

2. **Camp Model 205.** This model has an outer covering of very softweight foam with a filling of small shreds of foam. Available in sizes 1 to 7, size 1 corresponding to 30 inches and each one increasing 2 inches.

3. **Strodex Lightweight.** A kapok-filled breast prosthesis, available in small, medium and large sizes.

As part of a campaign to ensure that in time 'every mastectomee will be issued with a temporary breastform in hospital, the Mastectomy Association has recently introduced its own 'Mastectomy Cumfy'. This lightweight prosthesis can be washed and spin-dried, and the quantity of ICI-tested filling adjusted as necessary. Other points in its favour are the fact that it is being made by women in sheltered workshops or occupational therapy units, and the attractive price of around 30p. The Mastectomy Cumfy can be ordered direct from the Mastectomy Association (see page 121) but, naturally, the hope is that soon all hospitals will order this essential item from their own occupational units.

Incidentally, we recommend you wear a temporary breastform whilst travelling to and from your radiotherapy treatment. Because they are so soft and resilient, they also help to protect the area against accidental bruising.

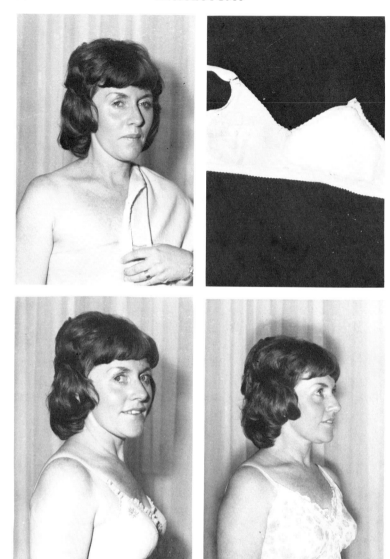

Photos courtesy of Nursu Wools

5. Stages in the cosmetic build-up of a mastectomee.

Selecting a Permanent Prosthesis

As far as the supply or purchase of a permanent prosthesis is concerned, remember it is not so much the degree of technical sophistication of the product itself that matters but a case of 'what is right for you'. We mention this because as someone on a limited income (a pensioner, perhaps), you may be baulking at the thought that you have to pay £50 to get 'the best' when, all the time, this may not be so in your case.

On the other hand, there is something very touching about the number of stories we have been told of how children have saved money to buy mum a 'super-duper' prosthesis for a birthday or Mother's Day or even Christmas. How very much such women must value their breastforms, and how very strong must be the family bond.

We have found that some women try two or even three kinds of forms before finding the make that suits them best of all, and back up a two-yearly renewal on prescription with a second item bought privately. Others have a 'wardrobe' of prostheses for different occasions, and that leads us to repeat one or two distinct points made to us by volunteers.

Granular. Usually the cheapest commercial form. Some claim it has the greatest movement; but its somewhat restricted shape does not readily lend itself to the addition of extensions to fill in the hollows of a radical mastectomy. Hard to the touch. Suitable for a sun-suit but not recommended for actual swimming.

Oil (sometimes referred to as 'liquid' or 'fluid'). Has good, fluid mobility and is therefore more natural to some women. Made in a wide size range. Fits into a pocket attached to your bra. Cannot be adjusted to match 'monthly fluctuations', and heat and perspiration or sea or pool water may discolour or deteriorate the foam base after a time. Natural-looking nipple.

Fluid/Air. Good, fluid mobility and very natural in wear. Absorbs body heat. Can be adjusted to match fluctuations in the true breast. Unaffected by extremes of temperature and chlorinated pool or sea water. Some women think its edges are 'a little hard'. Wide size range and, like the oil-type, it fits into a pocket built in to your bra.

Silicone. Puncture-proof and has an indefinite life. Very mobile and natural looking. Impervious to extremes of temperature, sea or chlorinated water. An important aspect is that it does not require a special bra. Absorbs body temperature in wear. Expensive, and some women reported very slight chafing as a result of perspiration in very hot weather. Wide size range but price varies according to size.

If you can afford to ring the changes you may feel that a wardrobe of prostheses is the ideal thing. Many women will tell you that there is nothing wrong with any prosthesis that a good bra will not solve, and there is a great deal of truth in this. Some honest corsetiere may tell you, in the nicest possible way that, single or double breasted, you've been wearing the wrong bra for years anyway – and then go on to prove the truth of her statement by creating a much better you. It does happen; and this is where a good corsetiere becomes worth her weight in gold.

If you are elderly, do not decide that you will do without a proper prosthesis without even looking into the situation. Quite a lot of older women have told us how very happy they have been to restore their figures to normal; and to the fashion-conscious woman of any age, a well-fitting prosthesis is vitally important.

A Morale Raiser

Women of all age groups have told us how their morale has been so uplifted by the fitting of the first prosthesis that they have wanted to run into the street shouting: 'Look at me. Look at me. I'm normal again.'

A few months ago a very beautiful woman (a former fashion model now almost fifty years of age) arrived at the fitting rooms of a local supplier, having been discharged from hospital that very morning. For two whole hours, and with the client's husband in attendance throughout, a conscientious corsetiere painstakingly fitted, adjusted, compared and readjusted various items of mastectomy apparel until the client's figure had been completely, undetectably restored. Fully dressed, the woman looked as beautiful as ever.

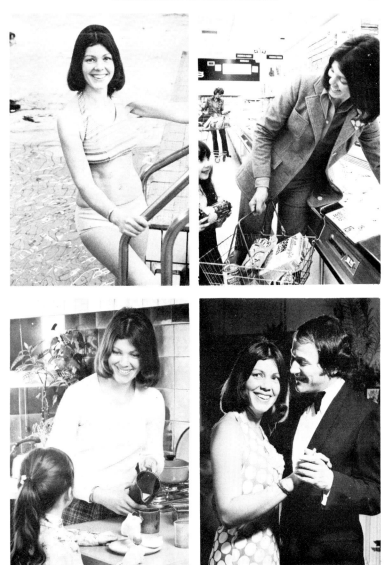

Photos courtesy of Ross & Hilliard/Patientcare

6. Total recovery. Ann Raine, 39-year-old teacher, had her mastectomy five years ago.

Realizing that the client was a perfectionist who might suspect bias in the husband's assurances that once again all was perfection, the corsetiere slipped away to return in seconds with an unbiased male from another department. The newcomer took a long, hard look at the elegant creature in the tight-fitting blouse and when invited to identify the artificial side of her figure was completely unable to do so.

The former model looked at the transparent approval in the young man's face: 'Now I know I'm all right', she said.

The key to your rehabilitation is the belief that soon, with the undetectable replacement of a few inches, you will be completely restored to normal appearance and completely normal life. You will still be the same woman. So believe it. The sooner you have thought yourself into that frame of mind, the sooner you will start to progress.

In time, a breastform becomes less of an extension and more a part of the person herself. Husbands, and the occasional 'unbiased male', can be seen to display very 'normal' assurances.

'When the dishiest man in the office smiled at me in that same old way, it didn't just prove something, it seemed like the best news I'd ever had.'

Don't spoil things by being so introspective that you fail to notice the unspoken compliment that can be such a morale booster.

Mastectomy Apparel in the USA

We have said that, commercially, Britain lags behind some other countries in its slow acceptance of mastectomy apparel as normal retail merchandise. American visitors will doubtless agree! But we should also add that commercial differences merely reflect the deeper and more enlightened attitude of American society towards the mastectomy subject as a whole.

The credit for this is due almost entirely to the work of one woman, Terese Lasser of New York, who, following her own mastectomy in 1953, began an educational crusade which ultimately swept America.

As the forerunner of many other Mastectomy Associations

and voluntary organizations throughout the world, the ACS Reach to Recovery Program founded by Terese Lasser has inspired an inestimable number of women to reach for and succeed in the recovery from cancer. Internationally, no other person has made a more significant contribution to this field.

Stimulated by Ms Lasser's self-help campaign and the recently revised Medicare scheme which allows breast prostheses and mastectomy bras to be claimed as legitimate medical expenses, American manufacturers and distributors remain in the forefront of technical innovation, presentation and service. And as the demand for more sophisticated and more feminine mastectomy products · has grown through voluntary organizations in other world markets, more and more of the sophisticated American-type products are being sold internationally.

Although present day American prostheses fall broadly into the same categories as UK brands, i.e. weighted and unweighted rubber/kapok; fluid and fluid/air; liquid and silicone gel; there are some subtle differences, not least in presentation and service.

The following detail on specific products may be useful to you as an American, or if you are currently living in America, or perhaps contemplating domicile in the USA. Prices tend to fluctuate and (as for UK) our quotes are intended as a rough guide only.

Foam rubber, unweighted and weighted forms, with acetate/satin covers of the type distributed by Madelon Louden, L.A., are available from many department/corsetry stores throughout the USA. Price: up to 15 dollars.

The Confidante fluid/air prosthesis (as described on page 42) distributed by Berger Bros., is widely available in stores throughout America. Price: around 45 dollars.

An alternative air and fluid filled prosthesis which is less expensive is the **Identical Form** marketed by Identical Form, New York. Price: around 30 dollars.

Brest Form by ATCO, **Miriam Gates** by Helene Barrie, **Tru-Life** by Camp International (described on page 43) and **Second Nature** by Jodee are all examples of liquid-filled prostheses in the 40-dollar bracket. **Brest Form** comes in both light and dark skin tones.

Companion by Airway Surgical is a sophisticated silicone prosthesis, basically the same type of product as the Poisette/Carefree breastforms now available in the UK. Under normal wear and care, it is claimed to have an indefinite life. Price guide: from around 85-120 dollars according to size.

An alternative silicone form at a lower price is the **Active** breast form by Stryker, a non-run silicone gel prosthesis with cleverly designed extensions under arm and upward towards the shoulder to fill in any areas where tissue has been removed. This form is also available in dark and caucasian skin tones. Price: around 75 dollars.

Most manufacturers (their full addresses are contained in the appendices to this book) supply a wide range of mastectomy bras and accessories including lightweight forms for immediate post-operative wear. Mastectomy Swimwear by Miriam Gates (Helene Barrie) is also available.

Please remember when writing to any manufacturer or distributor for further details that a stamped, self-addressed envelope brings a speedier reply.

We have gone on at some length – and we hope to some purpose – about the enterprise and innovation of American manufacturers and distributors. It is interesting to note that page 185 of the 1977 (spring/summer) Sears, Roebuck Mail Order Catalogue (the latest in our possession) is devoted exclusively to mastectomy needs.

The Sears Breast Prosthesis, we are told, consists of a liquid form plus foam rubber pad covered with nylon tricot. The form will easily withstand the pressures and frictions of ordinary wear and, as with a natural breast, it flattens when you lie down, assumes feminine contours when you stand and walk. The Sears prosthesis can be worn with almost any of your favourite bras or with the Sears specially designed bra also available by mail order. The pad is available in two shapes, one for simple and one for radical mastectomy. The prosthesis costs 40 dollars and the pad 5 dollars.

6. The Build Up:
Temporary and Home-made Prostheses

Though most modern mastectomees prefer to buy commercial prostheses, there are still some who prefer to make their own. And, contrary to what some people may think, not all the women in this do-it-yourself category do so from ignorance, as used to be the case in the Bad Old Days (not so old and faw away, actually) when the surgeon's stock reply to 'What shall I do to fill out my bra?' was often 'Oh, stuff a few old stockings in it.'

Judging from comments made by our research volunteers in every age group, there are women who have tried commercial prostheses and then decided to 'go one better' by inventing and improvising to suit their own requirements. These women are usually clever with their needles, are natural 'innovators', and are in a minority. This short chapter is devoted to those of you who may be in that minority group; and to those of you who may need to devise your own temporary bra-filler in areas where a commercially made lightweight is not readily available.

Protecting the Scar Tissue
Remember, even if you do not feel the need of a temporary form for cosmetic reasons, thought should be given to this practical fact: some sort of 'padding' acts as a buffer-zone to knocks and bumps in the same way as a bumper does on a motor car. Your scar tissue will be tender for some time; don't subject it to more stress than is necessary.

Scarves and handkerchiefs of pure silk are soft and kind to the skin, and stuffed into a bra give a natural (if temporary)

line. Some mastectomees have told us with pride and nostalgia
how they have used old family heirlooms for this purpose – silk
scarves that had been treasured by several generations for
various uses as the edicts of fashions changed.

Your normal bra may be too tight and/or too abrasive to
your scar tissue for a while after surgery. If you can afford it, a
'Gentle Fit' bra that fastens in the front is a worthwhile
purchase; or if you are comparatively small, one of the new
elastic-net, all-in-one-piece bras may fit the bill. Don't fall
prey to the assumption that the kind of bra you have worn for
years and years is the only one now on the market. There are
new styles coming out all the time and only a qualified fitter
can really assess what is available and which of these would
suit your temporary and later your permanent requirements.

Fitting a Temporary Prosthesis

Fitters 'calling' in hospitals usually work in the area of the
Appliance Office but some enlightened hospitals allow
mastectomy fitters on to the wards. Without being a nuisance,
'seek and ye shall find'! And then, don't let that fitter go until
you have determined the full range of bras and prostheses
available through that hospital and through private purchase.

Don't be afraid to contact the well-informed. For example,
the Mastectomy Association may be able to arrange for a local
volunteer to supply a temporary prosthesis faster than the
GPO can convey one from the Association's Croydon
headquarters. Failing that, the chances are that the volunteer
will be able to give you some useful help or advice towards
constructing your own.

Home-made Invention

Ruth was a 40-year-old schoolteacher, who wrote telling Nancy
of her (then) recent 'invention':

> My surgeon told me to wait two or three months after my radical
> mastectomy before being fitted for a proper prosthesis. I was
> discharged from a private hospital only a week after surgery and
> since I had promised myself that I would walk out in my kilt, as it
> were, I had to do something about filling the empty side of my

bra. I used cottonwool, a handkerchief and six little safety pins to construct what I called my sculpture. As I'm size 34B it was really not very difficult. Sister reckoned that when I was dressed I looked bigger than when I'd arrived, which was true. I had made my sculpture a bit too big so had to build up the other side to match it. I could laugh at myself then, which would have been impossible even two days before.

Once home, I decided to face the world full-on right from the beginning, and I still chuckle at the startled faces of friends and neighbours who came to visit a sick person and found me 'no different from before the op'. I was always dressed during the day; tried driving the car the day after I came home; and set myself a daily programme of gradually building up my strength by extending my exercises and activities day by day.

Ten days after the op, my family doctor removed the last stitches and I celebrated by attending my evening lectures. The fact that it was winter was in my favour, as I could dress more bulkily; and although things still hurt me badly at times, no one else seemed to recognize any change in me. 'It's all a matter of attitude' my surgeon had said one day, when we'd been sitting talking together on my hospital bed. He was right, of course, and through a previous year of wide reading I'd come to that conclusion myself in regard to living in general.

I bought myself some smart new clothes – polo-necked sweaters, a long skirt, a tailored sports jacket, a two-piece suit – and these boosted my morale so much that I accepted every invitation that came my way, from luncheons to dinner dances.

In the middle of the fourth week my cobalt treatment started, and the following Monday I returned to teaching my class of eleven-year-olds, going on to radiotherapy treatment each afternoon after school. The first days were a tremendous challenge. I was sure that my cottonwool sculpture was going to slip, but soon a new routine established itself, which blended into the old routine and all seemed to fall into place. I don't think my students knew the nature of my operation. Those eyes are so critical; but they have been gorgeous.

Now the radiotherapy is finished for me and I just have to wait for my skin to recover and my oesophagus to settle down. I suppose the summer will bring its own challenges but I'm already planning now how I'll adapt my swimwear and sunfrocks.

My husband has been simply marvellous, saying that he loves

me just as I am, with one breast or six or none at all. My teenage
children, a son and two daughters, have been equally wonderful
and I felt very flattered when they turned up in hospital with their
boyfriends and girlfriends.

Many women have said they needed a size larger bra for at
least a few months after surgery. If they were previously a 36B,
for instance, they needed a 38B bra until the scar tissue had
healed completely. The manufacturers listed in the appendix
operate a 'made-to-measure' or 'made-to-fit' corsetry service
through corsetieres working from home, and this includes a
special bra range with 'built-in' pockets to take a prosthesis.
This service is also available on prescription or at a special
price to patients in many hospitals. Again, this is your cue to
discreetly ask the right questions.

Whether or not you require a larger size bra depends to
some extent upon what sort of incision your surgeon made. If
you had a horizontal incision, well up from the normal line of
the bottom of the bra, your usual garment may not be any
discomfort whatsoever. But for the woman who has had a
vertical incision, going beneath the bra line, then obviously a
tight-fitting band on this area would be aggravating.

Hints for Avoiding Irritation

A radiotherapist, who has made a long study of post-
mastectomy needs, gives these additional hints:

1. Wear your bra inside out if the seams irritate the scar
tissue.
2. If making your own pocket to hold a prosthesis, always
cut the material on the cross.
3. Avoid bras that are underwired. But if you had that kind
before surgery and want to continue wearing them, remove
the wire.
4. Avoid metal or plastic clasps on the bra straps of the
amputated side. If you cannot avoid them entirely, at least
have them much *higher* than usual.
5. Your old bras can be adapted for post-mastectomy use
by inserting a piece of wide elastic at the back; by adding a

piece of elastic to the strap or straps; or by adding a front fastener. Any corsetiere worth her salt would arrange these adjustments for your.

Medical Sheepskin

There have been some interesting developments in the use of medical sheepskin in the last few years. In Australia, a prosthesis made entirely of wool is not only popular but is also very long-lasting. And because its teased-wool filling is easily accessible, this Nursu prosthesis can be adapted to day-by-day changes in the size, weight and contour of the remaining breast. The advantage of a lambswool pad next to the skin is that it is kind to scar tissue and therefore can be worn earlier than all other types. The all-wool consistency adapts to weather changes, being warm in winter and cool in summer, and absorbs perspiration well. In some Australian states, where the Nursu form is made under licence on the premises of the fitter, it is tailored to fit the client's chest. It is, perhaps, the only prosthesis which can be said to be 'custom-made'.

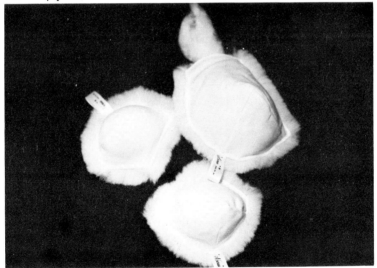

7. Three sizes of the *Nursu* prosthesis, the largest of which has been opened to reveal the teased-wool filling.

Before you rush off to Australia, we ought to mention that on examination the Nursu may not appeal to some of you as being 'fluid' enough in its movements for, say, dancing; and some people may feel that it is not weighted adequately. However, all things considered, in our opinion it is a first-class prosthesis with many, many advantages. And having said that, perhaps some enterprising distributor will now decide to import it and so save you from making that expensive trip to Australia. (Seriously, if you want to arrange your. own 'private' import, the address of the Nursu company is in the back of this book).

If you would first like to try a piece of medical sheepskin next to your skin, your chemist or surgical store may be able to obtain it for you. The skins come in various sizes and irregular shapes and you can cut off pieces from the jagged sides. If placed in alignment with your chest and arms the remaining piece could then be a great comfort to you in bed. One woman told us that she found a tiny pillow covered with a piece of medical sheepskin was a comfort as a 'prop' on her mastectomy side.

The most advanced type of medical sheepskin used in the UK is a material called 'Wolfix' produced by Morlands, the patent rights of which are jointly held by Morlands and I.W.S. This is produced by an ingenious method whereby the leather is removed from the wool and under heat and pressure the wool is bonded to a cotton backing. During this process the wool is not disarranged in any way. The result is virtually a sheepskin without a skin!

Wolfix is an ideal material from which to make either a temporary or permanent breastform as it absorbs a third of its dry weight in moisture without feeling damp. It can be washed repeatedly without any adverse effect and is light in weight. The material also allows air to circulate between the fibres, permitting the prosthesis to rise and fall naturally without any embarrassing adhesion to the body through natural moisture. No special bra is required; the addition of a few press-studs or a little Velcro to your normal bra will take care of any fear of the prosthesis slipping out. Incidentally, medical sheepskin is so kind to the skin that it is now used in many long-stay hospitals as a preventive measure against bed-sores.

Sponge Rubber
There are many stories of prostheses cleverly contrived from sponge rubber. A woman who was secretary to a top consultant described how she bought a green car sponge and cut it around until it was more or less the right shape. We should also mention that a sponge-rubber prosthesis is still available under the National Health Service and is also available privately from most suppliers at a cost of around £2.

Birdseed Filling
Birdseed was one of the first fillings used for breastforms. Though superseded by better materials in the eyes of most mastectomees and fitters, there are still women who swear by it. It is certainly one of the cheapest fillings, so experiment with it if you like.

This description from one of the birdseed devotees may help you. 'Fine birdseed has a lot of oil in it and it's slippery and moves with you. As I'm small, I need only a pound for both breasts. I cut out the cups from old bras, and slipstitch on a backing of cotton, leaving an opening through which I pour in the seed – just like stuffing a child's toy or a feather pillow. Then I tack or pin these "birdie bosoms" into a bra and find them very pliable and comfortable. To launder them, I just empty out the seed and re-use it later.'

Another mastectomee, a well-endowed nurse, wrote: 'I use a shaped bag with canary seed stitched into the lower area and teased lambswool in the upper section. Next to my skin I always wear a shaped piece of clipped sheepskin, the woolly side next to my skin, yet I cannot wear knitted woollen garments next to my skin. The medical sheepskin seems quite different.'

Shaping a Breastform
Home-made breastforms, just like commercial prostheses,

must be weighted to be successful. Women are ingenious with their weighting, too. Some use lead fishing weights; some use the round heavy button-like discs that are sewn into tailored curtains; while others use little balls of lead shot. Tiny bags of washed river sand, pebbles, dried peas and ball bearings have all been used at one time or another as weighting. We would stress though, that all these aids need to be worn in such a position that they do not cause abrasion to the skin.

Cups from old bras seem to form the basis, the *shape*, of many a home-made prosthesis. Much the same effect can be achieved if you cut a circle of stiff material about the size of the perimeter of your remaining breast, and then mitre it by making darts in the outside of the circle. Experiment with brown paper. Don't expect to get it exactly right at the first attempt. After all, you weren't taught to make false breasts as part of your school sewing lessons, were you?

But as women the world over are by nature and by nurture good at improvisation, and as necessity is the mother of invention, we are sure you will find a way to face the world with a convincing make-believe bustline. Even on a desert island!

7. Implants

Although operations for the insertion of internal prostheses, i.e. implants, have been practised in Britain for seven or eight years now, there is still a great divergence of opinion in the medical profession as to their true merit. Firstly, we must make it quite clear that not every mastectomy patient qualifies automatically; implants can be used only in certain, straightforward circumstances. Recent media comment on cosmetic figure changes and articles specific to mastectomy implants may have triggered off ideas in your mind about the possibility of an implant. All we would say is, before building up your hopes check with your family doctor or your surgeon that you are *physically* eligible, and then involve yourself and your husband in a full discussion of the pros and cons of the operation before going ahead.

If you want to talk to someone who has had implant surgery, then contact the Mastectomy Association who will put you in touch with a volunteer.

A Successful Implant

Jean is a 39-year-old Leicester housewife who had her mastectomy some three years ago. Following her post-mastectomy radiotherapy course, Jean wore an external prosthesis recommended by her hospital and soon resumed an active life. However, she still longed for the things she 'couldn't have':

> More than ever before, I longed to wear deep-plunge neck lines, bra-less dresses and so on; or at least to have the chance of

wearing them. I got in touch with the Mastectomy Association, the organization run by Betty Westgate to give help and comfort to breast cancer patients, and asked Betty if she knew anything about implant surgery. Betty knew a hospital in Birmingham that was doing the operation and advised me to try to get a referral there. Imagine my delight when a few weeks later my appointment with the hospital surgeon was concluded with the words 'Yes, I can give you back your cleavage!'

What's more, it was to be done on the National Health! Knowing this, I expected a wait of at least two years but somehow I struck lucky and within weeks I had been sent for.

No one can imagine the thrill of waking from the anaesthetic more or less symmetrical again and since then the boost to my morale has been tremendous, simply knowing that I can go bra-less if I want to and wear the lowest of neck-lines.

There is no doubt that Britain leads the world in this type of surgery and women travel from all over the country to be operated on at this famous Birmingham hospital.

It is to be hoped that in time, with more sophisticated methods of cancer detection and a wider knowledge and usage of fast developing surgical techniques, there will be less and less need for drastic surgery – thereby providing the opportunity of safe and effective implants for all who desire them. When that happens, we shall have reached an important stage in the psychological war against cancer.

Here is an opportunity for us to stress the importance of self-examination techniques to be carried out regularly by all women; as we have said before, cancer is no respecter of persons and it is clear that the sooner it is detected the more can be done. Jean's case is an example.

Self Examination of the Breast

It is to your advantage to examine your breasts regularly at the same time each month, e.g. the day after your period ceases. If you have passed the 'change of life', do this the first day of each calendar month.

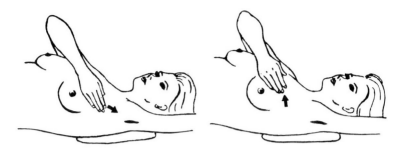

Examine the upper part of the breast, including the armpit, then the lower and central parts of the breast.

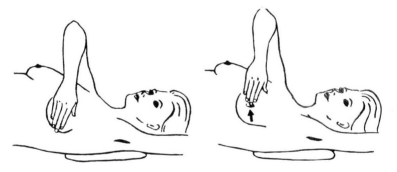

With your right hand, examine the whole of your left breast, as shown in the diagram, starting at the armpit. The left hand should be used if examining the right breast.

It is important to use the flat of your hand, keeping your finger tips held tightly together, making sure that the finger tips, the most sensitive part of the hand, follow the same path as the flat of your hand.

Should you find a lump in the breast (or any of the following 'warning signs') which was not present last month, go to your doctor and say 'I have a lump in my breast' or 'There is something wrong which I was not aware of last month'.

Warning Signs

Tell him carefully what difference you have noticed, and ask his advice. Through lack of knowledge some women only report to their doctor when a lump or swelling in the breast has been present a long time. The following points may be 'warning signs' that something could be wrong.

1. A lump or swelling in the breast.
2. Pain in the breast, not confined to the time just before a period.
3. A stained discharge from the nipple, or skin trouble around the nipple, or a 'pulling in' of the nipple.
4. An alteration in the appearance of the breast, e.g. dimpling or puckering of the skin.
5. A change in shape or size of one breast, compared with the other breast, which has occurred during the month.

You could show this chapter to your friends and encourage them to examine their breasts each month.

(The above instructions are available in pamphlet form obtainable from either the Mastectomy Association or Ross & Hilliard, 33 Albert Square, Dundee, and can be supplied in bulk to organizations willing to distribute them).

8. Arms and Exercises

Except in the rare cases where some complication makes exercise immediately after surgery inadvisable, it is best to start regaining mobility as soon as possible. This current theory contrasts with the old idea of leaving the arm immobile for a week or more, or even of strapping the arm to the patient's side.

If your surgeon has not raised the subject of arm movement within the first few days of surgery, make a point of asking him:

(a) if he recommends a particular form or range of exercises – some surgeons have a strong interest in this field and some may even have their own 'prescribed' exercises;

(b) if there is any reason why you must *not* begin exercises;

(c) if there is a staff physiotherapist who can attend you;

(d) and, if not, if he would mind your asking senior nursing staff for advice.

You might well find that the nursing staff have already been given the responsibility for advising you and will do so without prompting. The set-up varies from hospital to hospital.

At some of the larger hospitals, physiotherapists will call on mastectomy patients as a matter of routine but in others calls are made only if the patients (through the surgeons) request it. The opinions of surgeons may vary too, some feeling that early guidance on arm mobility is desirable and others that only common sense is necessary. We venture to suggest, though, that a woman's natural apprehension at how *much* she can do during the early days of recovery is an added emotional burden. 'No one told me just what I could or should do with my arm. It worried me. Was I doing enough? Was I doing too much? Was I trying to use it incorrectly? I would have welcomed more advice.'

Many women find that their shoulders ache for several weeks after surgery. They describe it as a nagging pain similar to toothache. As your muscles return to their normal strength, the shoulder pains will disappear, just as backache caused by lying in bed will ease when you re-use those muscles.

Using the Arm

As soon as possible, try to do your own hair, dress yourself, and do some crochet or knitting. A physiotherapist who has made a study of this suggests that the movements of crochet are more helpful than those of knitting; but not every woman has learned to crochet, whereas most can knit.

A woman who had a breast removed twenty-two years ago, told a touching little story. She was not a crocheter by inclination, yet had learned as a child. When she was advised to take it up again as post-operative therapy, she began making a cardigan for her baby daughter. By the time she had only half-finished it, her arm had regained good movement and she put the garment 'into moth-balls'. That daughter is now expecting her first child and the grandmother-to-be has brought out the cardigan to complete it. She says her hopes for the future were not very rosy when she packed that garment away twenty-two years ago, but here she is as fit as a fiddle and eagerly anticipating the birth of her first grandchild.

Women with young children, by the way, usually seem to make the quickest adjustments to breast surgery, both physically and emotionally. A small child needs constant physical attention, and a mother can't 'nurse' a stiff arm for long. It is forced into constant use; and that appears to be excellent therapy for it. Conversely, the middle-aged mastectomee, who is coddled and fussed over on her return home, takes longer to regain her arm mobility. Fortunately some husbands and sons realize the importance of exercise and a number of women have told us how the menfolk in their families have stood over them with Gestapo-like demands to 'let me see you do your arm exercises before I leave for work.'

It sometimes *hurts* to get the arm back to full mobility and this is where the encouragement of someone else in the family can be of immeasurable help. Just remember that any training hurts. If your son begins to do a two-mile run every morning to train for the football season, his muscles will hurt at first, won't they? Similarly, in training that arm back into the full swing of life you will find that the longer you have left it dormant, the harder the training will be.

The following pictures show a series of exercises designed to promote full mobility of the arms.

When you go home from hospital, rearrange your kitchen a bit – not to make things easier for your arm (as many women do, thinking it is common sense) *but to make your daily tasks just a little bit harder.* Put frequently-used objects (like your coffee jar and tea caddy) up high, so you have to reach for them. And raise your clothes-line a wee bit higher each time you hang clothes. That s-t-r-e-t-c-h-i-n-g and r-e-a-c-h-i-n-g is good therapy for your arm. Betty's 'walking fingers up the wall exercise' (Chapter 2) is an excellent therapy that can be carried out at any time.

Take Up Swimming

Swimming is one of the best and one of the first sports you can return to after a mastectomy. Make sure that swimming is part of your routine. Most towns of any size have a heated swimming pool and if you can get to the sea, so much the better. Even before your scar tissue is fully healed, sea-bathing is beneficial as a healer and as an exerciser. Some authorities feel so strongly about the recuperative values of swimming in the sea that they advise their patients to go to the seaside for a week or so after leaving hospital – even if this means considerable expense and considerable inconvenience to the rest of the family. If you and your husband can go together, all the better. It will be a period during which you can readjust to each other as well as to your immediate post-mastectomy needs. Always check with your doctor first and if he gives the

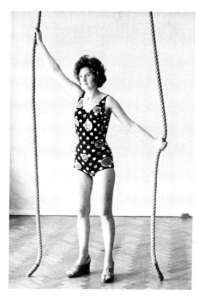

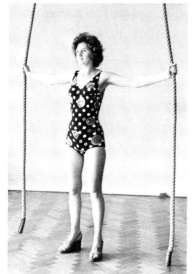

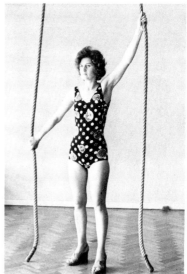

Photos by John Smith

8. Rope pulling exercise.

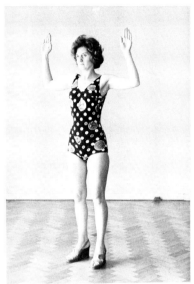

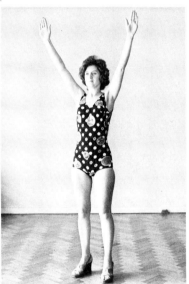

Photos by John Smith

9. Wall exercise.

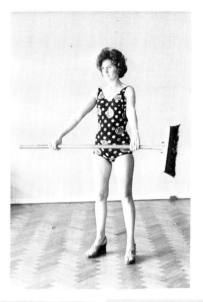

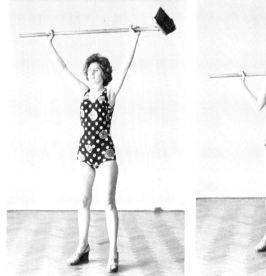

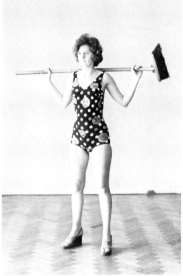

Photos by John Smith

10. Broom exercise.

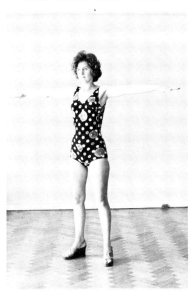

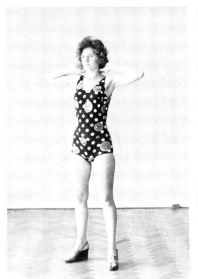
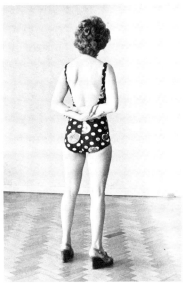

Photos by John Smith

11. Arm stretch and bend exercise.

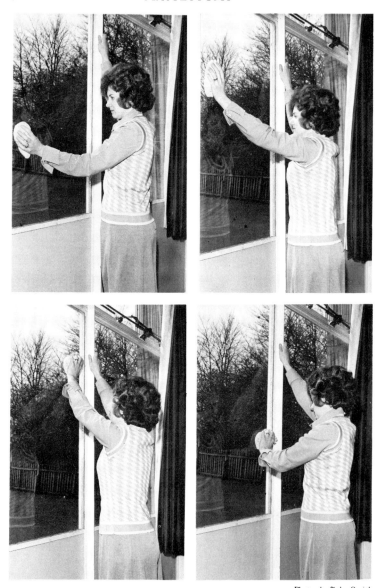

Photos by John Smith

12. Rotary polishing exercise.

'all-clear' (as a general guide for radiotherapy patients: not before eight weeks – you have to keep dry after radiation) set out in the knowledge that one week of seaside exercise and relaxation can be worth two weeks at home. If you really want to be alone together, there are stacks and stacks of seaside cottages, villas and flats to rent by the week or fortnight.

Another form of 'hydrotherapy' which every woman can undertake is to do arm exercises under a warm shower. Some like to do their exercises in time to music and certainly this can be a lift to the spirits as well as to the muscles – providing, of course, you can find the right kind of music.

Some Useful Activities

Women who have returned to typing jobs soon after their mastectomies also seem to experience a rapid return to full arm movement. Vera said: 'I had a breast removed when I was twenty-five, and I returned to work as a typist within three weeks. Then, two years later, I was expecting my first child and left work. It was only then that I began to have trouble with the arm and I really do feel that the typing had kept it supple. I hope it will be better again once I'm tending to the baby. In the meantime, I'm trying to work out exercises for it. My doctor wasn't much guidance when I asked him about it. He just grunted and said to use my common sense.'

Playing table tennis at home – a little more each day – is a happy, family exercise that has helped some mastectomees; while others have returned to golf or tennis or bowls within a month or so of surgery. You do not need sophisticated equipment for a scratch game of table tennis; just yourself, one other person, the dining room table and a couple of pieces of stiff cardboard to serve as bats. As the object is simply to keep the arm moving, the bat can be as big as a shoe-box lid. At least, you will not miss many shots that way. And if you can't find a partner, push the table against the wall and play off that.

One mastectomee, who drives a lot, told how she had trouble with her left arm until she happened to change from a car with automatic gears to one with manual gears. She felt that the gear-changing was good therapy for her arm, 'though it hurt like hell for a while', she added.

Problems with Dressing

While doing up back bra straps and zip fasteners may be impossible for a while after your mastectomy, don't think you will never achieve these gymnastics again. There are mastectomees who are afraid to try to do these things years after their surgery, yet there are many, many others who can soon clasp both arms behind their shoulders, or above their heads with the greatest of ease.

`If you would like to try an amusing but enlightening experiment, ask your husband or other male member of your family to don a bra and see if he can fasten it on his own back. He will think it's going to be a pushover until he has to get his hands into that position – then he grunts and groans and curses and carries on and finally admits it is harder than it looks. The moral is that you keep your muscles trained for those bra-fastening, zip-fastening motions every day, several times a day; whereas a man's apparel just does not call for them.

It would appear that more left breasts are removed than right breasts; yet right-handed women who have their right breasts removed have a subtle advantage over those who are right-handed but have their left breasts removed (or vice versa). This is due to the fact that a woman will force herself to use the hand and arm that are naturally her 'prime movers' and this in turn is good rehabilitation therapy for the muscles.

Watch Your Posture

Do be particularly conscious of your posture in the weeks following your mastectomy. There is a tendency to hunch over in much the same way as some girls do at puberty, or to lift one shoulder higher than the other. You may do either or both of these things quite subconsciously, yet neither habit is helpful to you physically, emotionally or cosmetically. Try to fight this pitfall by:

(a) asking your husband or someone else close to you to remind you gently when you are doing it;

(b) throwing your shoulders back in a deliberate and confident gesture;

(c) flexing your shoulders while waiting at a traffic signal, or watching television.

Remember: your arm movements are bound to be restricted initially but you must *attempt* movement; especially those exercises suggested by your doctor or physiotherapist. Do not try to force the arm too far too quickly but gradually increase the scope and level of activity day by day, week by week. By so doing, you will ultimately regain complete mobility of movement.

Should the arm become swollen, rest with the elbow above shoulder level by raising it on a cushion. You should mention the problem to your GP or hospital doctor.

Long-term Immobility

All the preceding comments in this chapter are about the ideal return to arm mobility soon after surgery. What about the woman who has not had help in hospital or from a radiotherapy department and who feels months or even years later that her arm is not as mobile as it should be? Can she be helped? Yes, she can, but of course the road back will be longer and more arduous.

If you fall into this category, have a chat to your family doctor about it. Say you would like to be referred to a physiotherapy department and just hope you do not strike a doctor who fails to realize just how helpful physiotherapy can be. Fortunately, there is an increasing awareness of the important role of the physiotherapist in the rehabilitation of the mastectomy patient and, indeed, increasing respect for the physiotherapy profession as a whole.

Lymphoedema

Post-mastectomy swelling of the arm or lymphoedema (pronounced limfedeema) can occur to greater or lesser extent in some but not all patients. To attempt to gloss over the incidence of it would do nothing to improve the distressing situation for those women who already have the condition and even less towards preventing it.

The incidence of lymphoedema is considerably lower than it used to be because of a better understanding of some of the causes. Yet we have been amazed at the number of letters from women depressed by this after-effect.

The last thing that we want to do is to alarm you; but we promised to tell you the possible problems. Sadly, this business of swollen or inflamed arms is still one of those problems and we hope the following set of questions and answers will help you understand lymphoedema and cellulitis in a positive way. Knowledge is power. Ignorance means fear.

Q. Does every woman who has a breast removed develop a swollen or inflamed arm on that side?

A. *No.* The incidence seems higher than acknowledged by some authorities but it is by no means inevitable.

Q. Are there any predisposing factors?

A. Yes. Women who have had radical surgery with the removal of lymph nodes are the most prone, while radiotherapy also tends to increase the tendency. Though rare in women who have had simple mastectomy with no subsequent radiotherapy, it is remotely possible; and elementary, common-sense precautions should be observed by all mastectomees.

Q. When could swelling and inflammation occur?

A. Almost any time after surgery. Swollen arms can occur many years later; but usually through ignorance of simple preventive measures.

Q. What are those measures?

A. 1. Make every effort to avoid injury to the hand and arm, which do not have as much protective mechanism to infection as non-mastectomees' have; or, indeed, as your other hand and arm have.

2. When gardening, always wear gloves. Mastectomees seem particularly prone to problems following scratches from rose or similar thorns.

3. If you get a splinter in your hand – and particularly if it is under a fingernail – have the splinter removed by a doctor if necessary, in the hope that you can prevent the onset of infection. For good measure, the doctor may also prescribe a course of antibiotics.

4. Try to avoid 'poisoned quicks' but if you do develop one, do not neglect it. Early in your post-mastectomy period, make an appointment to see a manicurist. Ask her to teach you correct nail care. Your chemist, too, has preparations for the prevention and treatment of poisoned quicks. Pamper your hands more than you have in the past. They could be your key to avoiding a swollen arm.

5. If you develop any form of infection in the hand or arm of your mastectomy side, go to your doctor *immediately* and ask for help. Failure to do this *can* cause later swelling of the arm (though, of course, many mastectomees could escape time and time again). We believe in: 'It is *better* to be *safe* than *sorry*.

6. *Never* let anyone take blood from the arm of your mastectomy side and likewise do not allow an injection to be given in that arm, or a drip connected to it other than on the authority of a doctor who has full knowledge of the facts of your case. Have your blood pressure taken on the other arm, too. In the case of bilateral mastectomees, always have these things done on the lesser side of the two. For instance, many bilaterals have one radical mastectomy and one simple. In such cases, always offer the arm of the 'simple' side. Or discuss with your medical team the alternative of using a leg. It would not be the first time.

Q. Can anything be done to prevent needles being put into my arm while I am unconscious?

A. Yes. Regardless of how long ago your mastectomy was performed, enrol now with Medic Alert Foundation (International). If your doctor or hospital does not have application forms, write direct to Medic Alert at the address given in the back of this book. When making out

Medic-Alert Membership Application
Send to: Medic-Alert Foundation
9 Hanover Street, London W1R 9HF

Full Name ....
(Block Letters)
Mr/Mrs/Miss ....

Full Address ....
(Block Letters)
....

Optional Next-of-kin, relative, etc.:
Full Name ....
(Block Letters)
Mr/Mrs/Miss ....

Full Address ....
(Block Letters)
....

TELEPHONE ....
Remittance enclosed herewith:
* Bracelet or Necklet:
  £4.50 + VAT .36   Total £   4   :   86
  Additional engravings (inc. VAT)
       11p each   £   :
* Delete as necessary   Total: £   :
Postal Orders and Cheques to be made payable to
'Medic-Alert Foundation'.
Signed ....
(Applicant or Parent)
Doctor's Name ....
(Block Letters)
Doctor's Address ....
(Block Letters)
....
....Tel:...................
DOCTOR TO SIGN OVERLEAF

Place X in box for size
of bracelet required | 6½ ins. | 7½ ins. | 8 ins. |

TO BE COMPLETED BY DOCTOR

Please place X in box
opposite engravings required

GROUP I PRE-EXISTING CONDITIONS: e.g.
- ☐ Diabetes
- ☐ Epilepsy
- ☐ Bleeding Disease
- ☐ Sickle Cell Disease
- ☐ OTHER ....
  (Block Letters)

GROUP II MAINTENANCE DRUG THERAPY: e.g.
- ☐ Steroids
- ☐ Blood Pressure Drug
- ☐ Anticoagulant
- ☐ Antidepressant
- ☐ Anticonvulsant
- ☐ OTHER ....
  (Block Letters)

GROUP III ALLERGIC TENDENCY: e.g.
- ☐ Penicillin
- ☐ Aspirin
- ☐ Insect Stings
- ☐ Serum (e.g. A.T.S.)
- ☐ OTHER ....
  (Block Letters)

GROUP IV MISCELLANEOUS CONDITIONS: e.g.
- ☐ Pace-Maker in situ
- ☐ Heart Valve Replacement in situ
- ☐ Contact Lenses
- ☐ Renal Dialysis Patient
- ☐ OTHER .... MASTECTOMY LEFT
  (Block Letters) SIDE. NO NEEDLES OR BP

If your doctor considers that additional information and
medical history to be necessary in an emergency,
this should be recorded him on the blank sheet
opposite for filing with Medic-Alert Foundation.

Doctor's signature ....

**DOCTORS ADDITIONAL COMMENTS
FOR FILING AT EMERGENCY H/Q**

Patient's Name   PATRICIA ANN SMITH

MASTECTOMY LEFT SIDE. NO NEEDLES

OR B.P. IN THAT ARM.

Doctor's signature ....

13. Example of Medic Alert Membership Application.

the form, use the words 'Mastectomy right (left) side. No needles or b.p. that arm' as shown in the illustration.

For a small fee, Medic Alert will issue you with a wrist bracelet and a personal identification folder. Once Medic Alert has your problem on file, doctors/police/ ambulance men/hospital personnel can 'phone a central registry and get full information by quoting the code on the inside of your bracelet. And through affiliated organizations, the service is recognized world-wide.

The once-only enrolment fee is cheap insurance that your arm will be treated with respect even if you are unconscious. Outside Britain, we know of a woman who had an injection into her affected arm while under anaesthetic many years after her radical mastectomy. Her resultant swollen arm has prompted her to take legal action in the hope that the case will help other women by drawing attention to the unnecessary distress caused through negligence or thoughtlessness.

Q. Can anything be done for women already suffering from long-standing lymphoedema.

A. That is a very difficult question, because medical opinion varies so much. Our advice would be to try the following measures:

1. Ask your doctor if he would consider referring you to the physiotherapy department of your local hospital, or consider recommending you to a private physiotherapist. Some physiotherapists are more skilled in this particular work than others and you must never go privately to a physiotherapist without first obtaining the approval of your doctor.

We recommend that you use only physiotherapists who are State Registered/Members of the Chartered Society of Physiotherapists (SRP/MCSP). As well as teaching you the correct massage and exercises, some doctors/physiotherapists have special equipment which they use in the treatment of lymphoedema. Such treatments (see illustration) can prove extremely beneficial. (Remember: never embark on any course of

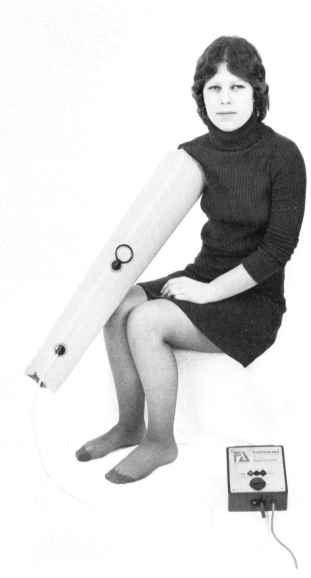

14. Flowtron intermittent compression system.

private treatment without medical approval. Do not attempt to purchase 'machinery' (pumps, etc.), with the idea of administering your own treatment WITHOUT THE SPECIFIC APPROVAL OF YOUR OWN DOCTOR; it might just be an expensive way of creating further and more lasting problems).

2. *Use* your swollen arm. There is a natural tendency to 'nurse' it too much and to hide it from sight. We should add that, though most physiotherapists and doctors agree that the arm should be used, there are other physicians who feel it should be rested; so ask your own medical team about it.

3. *Elevate* your arm as much as possible. While sleeping, try arranging a pillow on either side of you, so that whichever way you lie, your swollen arm is raised.

Some women have told how they have controlled their lymphoedema by having a simple pulley erected by their beds. Husbands and sons are good at improvising such gadgetry. One pulley-gadget we heard of had the arm strapped lightly to a cricket bat padded with lambswool! Care must be taken that the blood to the arm is not impeded; and you must also be able to move freely. A physiotherapist or a nurse would be able to instruct your husband/son in the elementary principles of a block and tackle.

4. A surgical supplier could sell you an elastic sleeve as illustrated (in certain circumstances, you may be able to get one prescribed).

In milder cases of swelling, this sort of therapy can be quite helpful. Similarly, crêpe bandaging (at least by night) helps some women. Talk to your doctor or pharmacist about it for there is a wide variety of elasticized bandaging now available. Another mild but readily tolerated 'sleeve' can be made from a disused support-hose, even if it has a small hole or two in it. Always elevate your arm for five to ten minutes before applying an elastic sleeve or bandage. And remember: like bandages anywhere, a bandage or sleeve which is not

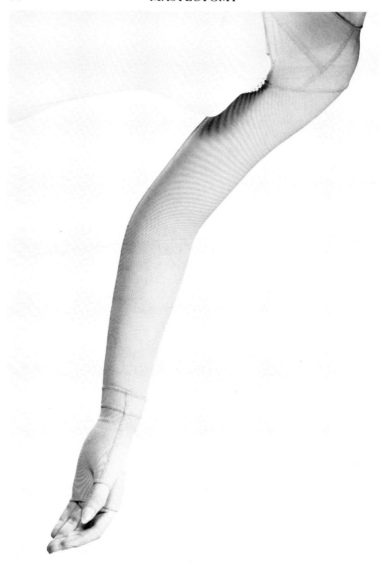

15. A Lymphoedema sleeve.

properly applied can cause oedema below the terminal end of the bandage – so make sure you get some instruction on how to apply it.

5. A hard oedema can sometimes be softened by the correct form of massage. Ask a physiotherapist to show your husband (or daughter or son or mother) how to do this.

6. In some extreme cases of lymphoedema, surgery is sometimes performed on the arm. Though surgery can bring about a successful reduction of swelling in some arms, you would be well advised to talk over all the pros and cons with your family physician as well as the surgeon.

Let us hope that with a knowledge of the precautions you should take and a practical approach to the subject, you will avoid developing any marked arm swelling or inflammation. We can assure you that the majority of women do escape lymphoedema and cellulitis, but insurance in the form of simple precautions is well worth while. After all, not many of us ever have our homes burnt to the ground, yet most of us take out relevant insurance policies in case of such an exigency.

If you do experience arm problems and they do not respond to treatment, try to take consolation from the philosophy of an Australian with a jovial smile and a zest for life, but also with a very swollen arm and hand.

'Nancy,' she said, 'this arm's a terrible nuisance, but when I realize I would have died if my breast and lymph nodes hadn't been removed so long ago, well ... this is a small enough price to pay for *life*.'

9. Radiotherapy

Contrary to what you may hear from second-hand rumours, radiation treatment need not be a period of fear and trauma. Before giving you a few hints on what to expect and how to make it interesting and challenging, let us explain that not every mastectomee goes on to have radiotherapy. Whether you do or not rests with your surgeon, who will take many factors into consideration. The majority of women are prepared to accept the surgeon's final decision on this matter, just as they accepted the surgery itself; but a minority feel compelled to question the wisdom of it. That is all right if you go about it sanely and quietly. Most surgeons would be only too happy to explain to you and your husband why they feel radiotherapy is advisable, and if you are still not convinced, they may even call in a second opinion to help you.

Don't feel 'cheated' if your surgeon tells you that radiotherapy is not indicated. It does not mean you are any less important, or that your surgery was any less necessary, or that your prognosis is not good.

Remember: radiotherapy is recommended in order to be absolutely sure that treatment of some cases is complete, but in many patients this is not necessary.

If you fall into the category of not needing radiotherapy, then just skip the remainder of this chapter.

What to Expect

On your first radiotherapy visit, you will probably be seen by one of the seniors in the department. He or she will explain the routine. Try to listen intelligently. If you allow yourself to become too tense at this time, feeling 'this is going to be an ordeal', you may miss out on the opportunity of getting to know this senior person. Remember, if you have any doubts and problems during the course of your treatment, this, logically, is the person you would ask to see again.

There are different forms of irradiation just as there are different forms of surgery, and it is not our place to differentiate. The duration of treatment varies from patient to patient. While the equipment used may also differ in minor points, the basic function is the same.

The following illustrations will give you some idea of what radiotherapy equipment looks like. We decided to include these preview pictures because, despite preparatory chats with the radiotherapist and past experience of various items of 'hospitalware', there are some women to whom the sheer size and scientific appearance of this equipment causes some apprehension when it is first sighted.

What is Radiotherapy?

Words without explanation are in themselves instruments of fear and to some women the scientific term 'radiotherapy' (popularly linked with cancer) sounds frightening; even though the same women have learned to accept the term 'X-ray' without getting alarmed.

When radiotherapy is simply defined as 'treatment of disease with X-rays or other forms of radiation' it immediately becomes less frightening.

You may hear of a variety of possible 'side effects' of radiotherapy treatment. Some women do experience certain sensations, a subject which we will return to later in this chapter, but often these are purely a by-product of unwarranted concern about the nature of their treatment.

Janet (Chapter 4) had been warned that the treatment might be unpleasant, 'but throughout I held on to the conviction that I was winning over cancer. Light meals, rest at the proper times and at no time was I sick.' That simple statement exemplifies the right attitude.

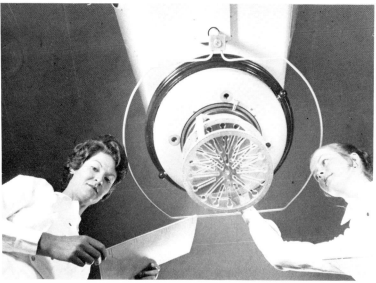

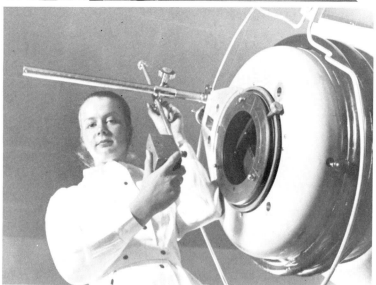

Photos courtesy of the Peter MacCallum Clinic
16. Radiotherapy equipment.

Psychological Reaction

Nevertheless, simply because no two humans are exactly alike, the psychological reaction to radiotherapy varies from patient to patient. Your reaction to being left peacefully alone and in no discomfort with 'the machine' will depend on your basic personality; for this is a time, rather like being under the dryer at the hairdresser's, when you are 'turned-in' upon your resources. (Some women despise their own company anywhere at any time, while others relish solitude anywhere anytime). Many women have told us how they passed the time while lying motionless under the machines. They counted seconds; or recited poetry; or sung quietly; or composed poetry; or recalled a favourite experience; or recounted cherished family memories; or relived a holiday; or prayed; or mentally redecorated their homes; or replanted their gardens; or planned a new wardrobe for the coming season. Any number of mental gymnastics have met the challenge of that Aloneness. One happy and very homely woman said she spent her time under what she termed The Thing, recalling old nursery rhymes to teach her young grandchildren. Another much younger woman confessed to reliving the same favourite experience at each visit!

Although you may feel alone while undergoing radiotherapy, you are not really. There is always a highly trained technician watching you from the control room; and there is always some method by which you can communicate with her if necessary. Some clinics may have taped music to play to you, but if you would rather be perfectly quiet, say so and the music will be turned off.

In speaking of her radiation treatment, Jean told us: 'They were fabulous to me. Initially, the consultant spent time in explaining basically what the treatment was all about and the technicians were among the kindest, friendliest people I have ever met. There was never anything forced or artificial about their attitude. Seemingly without trying, they always appeared naturally friendly and helpful and towards the end of my treatment it was so much like calling on old friends. When it finally ended, I really missed seeing them.'

For Jean, radiotherapy was what *she* and Leicester Royal Infirmary made it. Leicester RI, take a well-deserved bow!

Side Effects

You will not see, smell or feel a thing while you are under the machine. Before each treatment, however, you will probably be marked with a dye that can be a bit devastating to some fabrics. As the treatment progresses, you may (but by no means necessarily) develop a side effect or two. These can include nausea, tiredness, a sore throat or skin irritation. If you do develop any symptom, for goodness sake don't worry about it, as some women have told us they have done, and fear you have developed cancer in another part of your body. That is the fear that can inhibit your recovery and adjustment so *don't bottle it up*. Talk it out. Mention the symptom to one of the staff members at the radiotherapy clinic and they will be able to put your mind at rest and possibly give you something to alleviate the slight side effects. Many, many women go right through their treatment without any relevant side effects whatsoever.

Most people, though, do become tired. You may have to travel quite a distance and the travelling plus the treatment may eat into the days just when you are trying to resume the normal routine of caring for your family. Try to plan a rest for a while after your return home from treatment. Relax. If things do not get done today, then maybe tomorrow – or the next day – or next week. Keep as active and busy as you are able to; but don't drive yourself beyond your tolerance. Rome wasn't built in a day.

Emotional Impact

This could also be a period when the full impact of your mastectomy hits you emotionally. Most radiotherapy clinics are aware of this, and welcome questions on any aspect of rehabilitation. In this respect, you are more fortunate than the women who do not have radiotherapy and who, except for an occasional check-up by the surgeon, lose touch with the medical and paramedical services when they leave hospital.

Another good reason, we think, for becoming a member of the Mastectomy Association is that you are never out of touch.

If you want to take a husband or daughter or close friend with you for the first few treatments, you will not be the first to do so. You may wish to travel to the hospital in your own car; if you do so, check up on parking arrangements before setting out. With some hospitals, you may be able to arrange to be collected and taken home by ambulance-minibus at set times. However, as time goes by, try to use public transport for your trips to the clinic. This has two main advantages – firstly, your appointments can be made to suit you rather than waiting around at the clinic at peak times when the ambulance cars are arriving; and secondly, you will be getting out amongst ordinary, healthy people again; and that is of prime importance.

Do not shut yourself away. Life does go on. It is emotionally good for you to see it again, after being hospitalized and spending some of each day in a clinic where people are being treated for cancer. If you are well enough to undertake at least some public transport it is foolish to cocoon yourself away from all the vibrant colour of life by using private or special transport.

Finally, plan ahead for the day when your radiotherapy will end. You may think: 'Golly, I'll be so pleased not to have to go out every day.' Yet when the time comes, you could find that life seems a bit empty. Going to radiotherapy each day, seeing those cheery technicians, maybe making new friends amongst other patients, can all become a habit hard to replace unless you plan ahead for that sudden gap. Enrol for classes in a craft, or buy some material to sew, or stock up on some good books to read.

10. Clothes and Swimwear

'If everyone were able to put his troubles in a place for all to see,' goes an old saying, 'each one would prefer to keep his own burden.'

How true this is. It is also true that you will have specific troubles with your dressing in future, but don't we all? There are very few perfect figures and most of us have to be cunning in at least one aspect of choosing clothes. A friend of yours may have the burden of having large, swollen or in some way or another unattractive legs. Indeed, you may even be tempted to feel sorry for her – until it suddenly strikes you that, snazzily trouser-suited or in a lush evening gown, she has just succeeded for the umpteenth time in snaring the most attractive man in the room.

So, though you are going to have to be that little bit more cunning with your wardrobe too, you can rest assured that your problems are going to be no greater than anyone else's.

During our researches for this book, we found that the mastectomeees who are 'handy with their needles' have a distinct advantage over those who are inept or untrained in this basic feminine art. If you happen to fall into the latter category, give consideration to taking some lessons – not only in dressmaking, but also in the daily, down-to-earth adjustments and repairs to clothing that a clever needlewoman does as a matter of course. From such humble beginnings, whole new businesses have grown! At the very least, you might save yourself and your family some money.

If you happen to be good with your needle and you are

looking for a post-mastectomy interest, consider giving lessons to schools, Girl Guide Groups, young marrieds and so on. In other words, spread your talent around, it may be just the emotional stimulus that you (and perhaps some of your pupils) need at this particular time.

Shopping Problems

While some shop assistants understand the problems of clothes for mastectomees, there are others who are not only unhelpful, but who can cause unnecessary stress to a client by showing revulsion at the sight of any scarring or burning that may extend beyond the bra-line. We would therefore like to make a plea for all department stores and boutiques to make sure their applicable sales assistants have some tuition on the specific clothes needs of mastectomees in terms of intimate apparel and outerwear. Anyone wishing to arrange for such tuition should contact his or her nearest supplier of mastectomy apparel, asking if a trainer could be assigned.

To make sure that you are not offended by an insensitive or unqualified assistant, ask for the supervisor of the department concerned. Say: 'I've recently had a breast removed and would appreciate some help in selecting a new garment.' Don't mind adding: 'Do your assistants understand the situation?' We think it is a national disgrace that so many of them do not.

However, the approach we have outlined is far less distressing than to see horror registered on the face of an 'uninitiated' assistant when you undress. Or you could do some preliminary checking by telephone and so make your own little list of sympathetic stores. We can assure you that there *are* some very discreet and sympathetic shops and stores. We hope that, in time, branches of the Mastectomy Association will have lists to give to 'new chums'; the fact they are making constant enquiries as to what is good and what is bad may ultimately be reflected in the customer's loyalty to the store for mastectomy and other purchases; for such are our rights as consumers.

Choosing Styles

If you have a hollow above the bustline and/or in from the underarm (where the surgeon, in your best interest, removed some extra tissue) you will find that clothes have a tendency to 'fall into' those hollows instead of hanging properly. This can be minimized if your corsetiere has added some padded extensions to your bra in the relevant places and if you wear raglan sleeves whenever possible.

Plunging necklines and sleeveless styles can be embarrassing, particularly when you bend over or raise your arms, unless compensated for. Again, your corsetiere, surgical fitter, dressmaker, enlightened sales assistant or fellow mastectomee are the best counsellors. A minority of mastectomees avoid all low-cut frocks, but others wear these styles and still avoid revealing scars or indentations or parts of the prosthesis by the simple expedient of weaving some elastic thread through the neckline and/or armhole, so that the garment fits more snugly into the body. If much tissue has been removed from the outer axilla (underarm) you will have to make the personal choice between always wearing dresses with long or short sleeves or contriving to show only a minimum amount of the mutilation.

Some mastectomees find halter-style suntops are good at covering outer scars and depressions. These need to have broad halter straps sweeping up from the underarm. With such a style you would need to wear either a halter-neck bra to hold your prosthesis, or a pocket sewn into the outer garment.

Adapting Your Wardrobe

Buy a new garment or two as a morale booster by all means (red seems a favourite 'cheering-up' colour) but unless you have an unlimited budget, don't rush in and buy a totally new wardrobe. Most of your present clothes should be adaptable.

Add a contrasting inset here, take in a dart there, add a pocket or a ruffle or a cap sleeve somewhere else. Until you have complete confidence that your prosthesis gives you the right line and that your corsetiere has ensured it stays in place, avoid plain bodices. Distract the eye of the beholder away from the bust and on to trimmings such as collars, pockets, drapes, shoulder tabs, or even scarves. Chunky beads or cameos that sit at the base of the throat, shoulder brooches or anything else that raises the eyes above the bustline can be useful until you feel absolutely confident that you are 'undetectable'. Similarly, dangling ear-rings can help if you happen to have pierced ears and if you are the slightly flamboyant type who can wear that sort of thing. People will not 'size you up' nearly as much as you think they will.

Some small-breasted women find it beneficial to build up the existing breast to a size larger; and certainly your surgical fitter should ensure that your real breast is well-uplifted. It is no earthly good having a new, pert false breast if your real one is drooping down to your toes. Bilateral mastectomees (such as Kate, Chapter 4) have the opportunity, for the first time in their lives, of deciding what size bust they would like to have. Some choose a size or two smaller than was endowed by nature, but it is a mistake to decrease the size too much. Nature probably also gave you wide shoulders and hips and too small a bust-line then looks out of place.

Adding Prosthesis Pockets

While working or on holiday overseas, it will be harder for you to dress when the mercury and the humidity climb. A young woman from the northern part of Western Australia said: 'I cannot wear bras in the summer here, so I've made invisible pockets in most of my frocks where I can insert the prosthesis. This is easier if the dress has a front seam because I can then attach one side of the pocket-cum-lining to the centre seam as well as to the garment's side seam.'

At home or overseas, it is a good idea to sew a pocket into your nightdress or housecoat. The pocket can hold a prosthesis or other filling and so save the embarrassment of being seen without a bust. It also nips in the bud the unfeminine habit of clutching the gown beneath crossed arms – a gymnastic mannerish which is as uncomfortable as it is unattractive and futile. Add a pocket for a prosthesis to your bedjacket, too, so that if you ever have to go to hospital, you

can assume a normal appearance whilst sitting up in bed. You
would be surprised how often the fear of 'what will happen if I
ever have to be hospitalized again' has been expressed to us by
otherwise well-adjusted mastectomees. A similar fear is that of
being found by police or ambulance-men after an accident.
Policemen and ambulance-men did not actually come down in
the last shower, but if you happen to be worried about this
aspect of life in the future (and we all have our phobias of
some kind) then enrol with Medic Alert so that your bracelet
will give a subtle warning.

Nightgowns can have ruffles down the front; and you may
like to invest in a second 'temporary' breastform which can be
pinned or press-studded into your gown. These are available
from the major suppliers or through the Mastectomy
Association.

Swollen Arms

For mastectomees with swollen arms, clothing can present
specific challenges. Here, then, are some hints from women
who have learned to live with this condition.

1. As few ready-made clothes in your normal size will have
sleeves wide enough to fit over a marked lymphoedema, a
piece of material must be inserted to the under-sleeve. A
skilled fitter-corsetiere can show you what to do or may
even offer to make the adjustments in her workroom. Again,
the self-employed corsetiere is usually more prepared to
help than shops and stores. If you are a short person you
have an advantage, because a piece of material can be taken
from the hemline and inserted into the sleeves. If no such
'spare' material is available from an off-the-peg garment,
buy some contrasting braid or petersham ribbon. Add the
inserts to the upper part of the sleeve and to make it appear
part of the design, add a band of braid to the outer sleeve as
well.

2. Always make *both* sleeves large, then pad the sleeves of
the normal-sized arm with foam, and lift it a little at the
shoulder. This obviates the lop-sided look of having one arm
larger than the other.

3. Always test the 'stretch' of ready-made knitted garments to make sure they will accommodate the swollen arm without being restrictive.

4. Buy good, tailored clothes that will not date. Find yourself a top-class dressmaker who knows how to compensate for your swollen arm. She will be expensive, but if you choose your fabrics and style carefully, her garments will last far longer than cheaper off-the-peg clothes that do not fit you properly.

5. Join the Mastectomy Association and let the secretary know that you would like to exchange clothing hints with other lymphoedema members.

Swimwear

Finding the right swimwear for post-mastectomy needs has been a major problem to some women in the past. However, we understand that since this problem was first aired in the media some eighteen months ago, at least one key manufacturer is considering extending its range to include lines suitable for mastectomees.

The following models are from a wide range of swim and beachwear specially designed by Torplay, St Bees, Cumbria and available direct from them by mail order. Suits are fitted with pockets suitable for all types of prosthesis, so all you need to do is to write to them enclosing a stamped, addressed envelope and select your suit from the brochure and material samples sent to you. The style, material and bust size should be clearly stated on the order form and an alternative choice of material should be given where possible. Customer alterations to stock size garments can be undertaken at a small additional charge, necklines can be raised or lowered and sleeves put into certain styles. Support panels can also be inserted on request and skirts and trousers made in the same materials if desired. Prostheses specially recommended for swimming are also available.

The simple advantages of purchasing your mastectomy apparel in this way are in knowing that the style of the garment will be entirely suitable for your purpose and, of

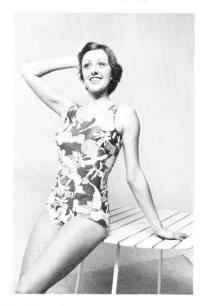

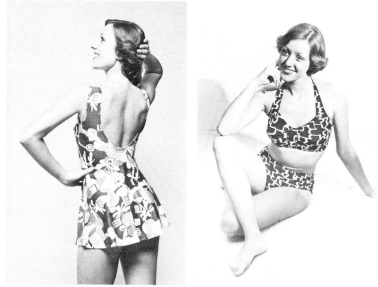

17. *Torplay* swimwear.

course, the over-all confidentiality of the service. Knowing that you can wear any particular garment with absolute confidence is vitally important at every stage of your rehabilitation.

Locally, you might discuss swimwear with your surgical fitter who most certainly will be tuned in to whatever new is happening in this field. She may even stock a few suitable lines herself and could also add the necessary prosthesis pockets for you, in those lines where such a pocket and/or prosthesis is not already part of the original design.

Adapting Swimwear

It is not always necessary to buy new beachwear. Once again, the woman who is handy with her needle can improvise some cover-up. One young mother who swathed a cover-up band of contrasting nylon from one shoulder strap down to the 'V' of her swimsuit created such a stunning Grecian-look style that the unsuspecting women of a local club copied it!

For small women an old fashioned foam 'falsie' (or 'bust improver') is probably adequate build up for swimming; but take heed that your prosthesis is securely fastened no matter what type you use. To have your bust suddenly floating upon the waters may be funny to some (Chapter 4), but could be far from funny for you.

Covered, foam-rubber bust improvers – like those shown overleaf – are inexpensive and available at many stores and corset salons.

Unless you are wearing one of the special 'swimproof' prostheses, you must remember to squeeze excess water from your prosthesis when you come out of the water. Failure to do this means that you will, at the least, dry out 'unevenly' (bang goes your secret), and excess salt or chlorine may shorten the life of your prosthesis. 'Old hands' tell us that getting rid of any excess water is easy enough to do if you pretend to be drying your face and neck under cover of the towel, and just exert extra pressure on your false breast.

As stated in the chapter on exercise, swimming is excellent post-mastectomy therapy, so go out of your way to have

swimwear you are relaxed in. A grandmother of no mean
years told how she had taken up swimming again after many
years because her surgeon advised it. Now she swims daily at
a heated pool and her husband and young granddaughters
share the fun of it with her.

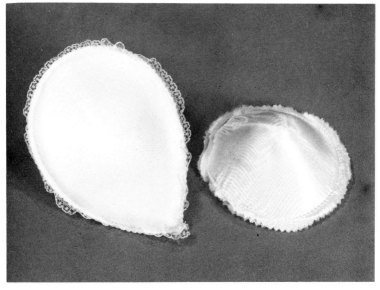

18. Bust improvers.

11. For Husbands and Families

The success of a woman's post-mastectomy adjustment is often in direct ratio to the understanding of her husband and family; so, in addition to passing references in other chapters, we have set aside this special section for busy husbands and families to read even if they do not have the time to scan the whole book.

It is not easy to advise a man on his attitudes to his wife's mastectomy, recognizing as we do that no two persons think or feel in exactly the same way. But we have spoken to many medical and paramedical people about it, and with husbands both separately and with their wives.

Jean's Story
For Jean (Chapter 7), the initial reaction was one of complete devastation; more than anything she needed the love and understanding of a good man.

To me it seemed like the end of the world. Thirty-six years of age, divorced, two children and only just engaged to be married. A mess. What were my chances now? After years of unhappiness, I had finally found the right partner; the ideal father for my two youngsters and someone they adored. Now, the discovery of two tiny cysts, no bigger than the size of peas (which three months before my doctor had described as 'nothing to worry about') seemed to have placed our whole future in jeopardy.

Despite my GP's assurances, I had gone on worrying about those lumps in my breast and now I was into a nightmare of tests that were positive, attending hospital for what we all thought was a minor operation only to find myself two hours beforehand signing a form that gave permission for removal of a complete breast 'if we find it's necessary'.

The doctors and nurses were kind and their obvious care and efficiency inspired confidence about the success of the operation itself. All that bothered me was the effect of the operation on the man that I and the children had learned to love so much. How would I explain the fact of losing him? God bless them, what could they do but blame me? I told myself over and over that I must understand if his revulsion was more than our relationship could take. I prayed that it wouldn't be.

The moment I came round, I knew from the surgeon's face that a complete removal had been carried out. 'You've done it – haven't you?' 'Yes,' he said, 'we had to.'

I cried until Brian came and told me that it didn't matter a damn and that it was the real me he loved and not just my breasts; and yet even when he left I wondered if he would come back the next day. But he did – every day – cycling ten miles on a pushbike in all weathers just to be with me and to hold my hand and to make me believe nothing had changed.

We were, if anything, even closer than before the mastectomy. I swore that one day soon I'd give him something better than a bike! We are, of course, married now. I could have understood if Brian had changed towards me. It would have been hard but I would have managed somehow; indeed, at one stage I'd resolved myself to it. But his love and understanding then and since have made my life so much more worthwhile, so much richer for the experience.

Jean and Brian; two very wonderful people. If you are reading this as a husband, or steady boyfriend, doesn't it make you proud of your own sex? As a father or brother, wouldn't you like to think your daughter or sister's husband would react in the same way as Brian did?

Compensating Factors

Fortunately, Brian is by no means alone. There was, for instance, the husband of a young bilateral mastectomee who said: 'I didn't ever consciously try to understand why I was first attracted to Sue. At the time I know her sexiness was a big draw and it probably wasn't until she lost her first breast that

I knew for the first time how much I loved the real Sue. The most important thing in the world became that she should *live*. A chap at the office, whose wife had a breast removed last week, asked me had I missed Sue's breasts. I almost laughed at him. Hell, of course you do, but the other thing – the getting closer spiritually, more than compensates. Or for me it does, anyway. Our sex life is better than it ever was.'

This positive factor knows no age barrier. A woman of sixty-three told us: 'Something good has come from my surgery because my husband and I are closer now than we've ever been before. This was our first real adversity and it taught us not to take each other for granted.' And a 28-year-old: 'My husband has been absolutely wonderful throughout. He saw the wound at its ugliest – all bruised with a row of green stitches marching across the ribs. Not then, or since, has he shown any revulsion whatsoever. We are even closer together than before the mastectomy.'

Another woman, who had had a mastectomy when her children were only three years and eighteen months old respectively, wrote: 'My husband has been marvellous all the way. I don't know how I could have coped without his understanding and love and patience. Whenever I'm tempted to be cross with him, even now so many years later, I just remember those worrying early days and my heart melts with humbleness.'

Poor Communication Between Partners

On the other hand, Evelyn (who has had her ovaries removed as well as a breast) wrote: 'My husband didn't appear to have any feeling. Eventually I asked him about it. He just grunted and said, "Of course I've been worried about you". I would have loved a few words of reassurance occasionally. He's never been demonstrative but at this he just seemed stony.'

Poor communication is a barrier to most aspects of readjusting to mastectomy, but nowhere is it more apparent than between marriage partners. If you have not communicated well with your wife in the past, it will not be easy to begin now; but please believe us when we say it is so necessary. Be brave. Say those words you may have thought 'sloppy' or unnecessary in the past. Not infrequently we have heard of couples where each partner thought the other had lost interest. The husband had thought he was doing the right thing in not making sexual advances to his wife. She, poor devil, had thought he was revolted by her 'mutilation' and so had not given any signs that her confidence needed the boost of knowing that her husband still desired her.

Vicious circles, unnecessary stress and suffering, all caused by *poor communication*.

Author Penelope Mortimer, best known for her *Pumpkin Eater*, wrote another novel called *My Friend Says It's Bullet Proof*. This book is about a sophisticated journalist who, during rehabilitation from mastectomy, is sent on an overseas public relations assignment with a lot of male colleagues. During the trip the heroine goes out of her way to make sexual conquests just to prove to herself that she is still woman enough to do so.

A strange sort of novel, you might say, yet every time we have recounted that story, we have been told by outwardly well-adjusted, 'respectable' mastectomees that it had struck previously unacknowledged chords. If only they were 'that type', they say, or if they were more sophisticated then they would like to prove to themselves that they could still 'get a man' just as Penelope Mortimer's heroine did.

Not that we want to encourage mass extra-marital soliciting by mastectomees, or to frighten you that your wife will be casting her eyes in other directions! We just tell the Penelope Mortimer story and its reactions to help you realize how very important it is that you reassure your wife of her femininity, especially if she has also had a hysterectomy and/or an oopherectomy. If you still desire her, *say so*.

Someone to Depend On

Most women appreciate one devoted lover in their husbands, despite the reaction to the Penelope Mortimer story. It is a comfortable feeling for man and woman to know that there is 'old faithful' – someone to depend upon – part of the reason for marriage. So many women have told us that if anything happened to their husbands they could not possibly face starting a close liaison with another man who did not understand about the mastectomy. Yet Jean and many, many others have remarried or married for the first time after losing a breast.

If your wife's chest and/or arm are still sore you will need to be particularly gentle in your physical approaches to her and each couple will need to make its own adjustments. Sometimes, it is as simple as changing sides. *Talk* about your problems, maintain a sense of humour, and a way through the woods will be found, maybe not at the proverbial drop of a hat, but given time and love and patience.

Social workers who have helped and supported women in cases where a mastectomy has been blamed for a subsequent break-up of marriage, observe:

(a) that most of these marriages were very shaky long before the mastectomy, and

(b) that the husbands who reacted badly to a wife's mastectomy were immature and unable to cope with stress.

A Vital Role

The husband can play a vital role in helping a wife to make a complete recovery following her mastectomy operation. The way *you* accept the effects of the operation can make a difference to the speed of her acceptance.

Extra caring will undoubtedly be welcome, coupled with the assurance that together you accept that the loss of the breast has no bearing on your continued relationship with each other.

When you see the results of the operation, deal with it in a normal and unemotional way. A positive remark can help, such as 'It's healing well' or maybe 'The surgeon has done an excellent job' or something along these lines.

Try to observe these guidelines:

1. Demonstrate your love in words as well as actions; but take care not to overdo the 'pity bit'. (Betty's story: '...

although he was always there to lean upon, he had the sense never to be over sympathetic to the point where it might detract from my own efforts to get back to normal.')

2. Talk to at least one of her medical team. If you would like to talk to another husband who has been through this mutual adjustment period, the Mastectomy Association, local cancer authority, or the hospital surgeon may be able to arrange an introduction.

3. Send some red roses to a blue lady; or take her some champagne.

4. Never show revulsion to your wife's scarring, and do not avoid watching her dress or undress or she will fear you are revolted.

5. Remind your wife about arm exercises. Go swimming with her if possible.

6. Encourage her to buy a good prosthesis. If necessary, make the appointment for her and metaphorically hold her hand by taking her for the fitting if she indicates she would like that.

7. Be careful of your jokes until you are quite sure they are not hurtful.

8. Never joke about – or discuss – your wife's mastectomy in front of other people.

9. Admire your wife's clothes and grooming. Buy her something pretty and feminine *yourself*. She will know instinctively if you have just sent your mother or secretary out for it.

10. Take her to a quiet, candle-lit dinner as soon as she is well enough. And/or the theatre if that is more her line.

11. Encourage her to take up some new, creative interest. Maybe start something new together – pottery, sailing, antiques, art, amateur dramatics, the list could be endless.

12. Remember that anxiety is as contagious as measles. Try to be contagious with serenity and hope rather than anxiety.

13. Make it your aim that your wife will be able to say, as others have said: 'I look normal, I am normal. I am happy.'

Help From Families

Much of what has been said to husbands is equally applicable to families, but if you are a close female relative you are at a disadvantage in the way you relate to your mother's/daughter's(sister's mastectomy. It is a 'bit too close to home' for comfort. Either you feel 'there but for the grace of God go I' or you have already had a breast removed and in reliving all your own traumas you unconsciously or sub-consciously bequeath them to your mother/daughter/sister.

You can, in fact, be an unexpected but positive hindrance to her rehabilitation. Even as a fellow mastectomee, you are likely to be ineffective as a counsellor to someone within your own family whilst remaining a godsend to a total stranger. Why that is we do not quite know other than that it fits in with other aspects of behaviour where we are clumsier with, less patient with and expect more from those closest to us than we do from total strangers. Furthermore, the new mastectomee's response to a female counsellor in her own family is often a low and reducing one in that she is only listening to 'old Marge rabbiting on the way she's always done' whereas a gentle, diplomatic stranger, has her credibility 100 per cent intact from the very start.

Although it does not always follow, just take heed if you are a female relative of a new breast amputee, because you will need to assess all your attitudes to this mother/daughter/sister to make sure you are not being over-anxious or over-sympathetic or over-hard or ostrich-like or just plain bitchy.

Male relatives (fathers/sons/brothers), on the other hand, seem to react instinctively in the right ways, and rarely hinder. In all our contact with many hundreds of mastectomees, we cannot recall having one single complaint about the attitude of a close male relative (other than husbands).

Problems with Female Relatives

If you are the mastectomee with a difficult mother/daughter/sister, try to realize that this is a common problem. Some female relatives are so ostrich-like, for instance, that they just refuse to acknowledge that the mother/daughter/sister has had a breast removed – as though the whole nasty business will go away if they ignore it. Not infrequently the patient is more calm about her operation and about the fact of cancer than her close female relative. Such a patient often finds herself giving an emotional lift to her female relatives. In small doses this can be all right, but just make sure if you are the mother/daughter/sister that you are not demanding too much from the mastectomee.

Do not overdo the you're-lucky-to-be-alive-bit, either. There will be times when the patient will wish she weren't and to have you harping like a Pollyanna-gone-wrong does not help the situation.

Muster all the subtlety, tolerance and tact that you can. Granted, your mother/daughter/sister may be irrational, moody, depressed and hard to please; but do not barge in with a bulldozer full of platitudes and think it is going to help. Let her lean on you a bit if she wants to, but do not become a permanent crutch. Refrain from narrating second-hand, gory experiences of other mastectomees.

Encourage the new breast amputee to take a fresh interest in her clothes and grooming; take her to the hairdressers or for a drive in the country; accompany her to radiotherapy if she seems to need support but make sure, first, that you are not encroaching on her husband's territory in any of these things.

Because male relatives, especially sons, somehow know instinctively how to relate to a new mastectomee and can be more objective in their outlook than the patient herself, her husband or her female relatives, we do not consider it necessary to give any specific advice in this area.

Practical Help

In practical terms, the whole family can contribute a great deal towards a woman's speedy recovery, by lifting heavy loads for her, helping with the ironing, the washing-up, making beds, and generally seeing that she does not become over-tired during the first few weeks after her return home.

You will find that these extra considerations pay dividends, the patient will feel more relaxed within the family circle and this in turn can lead to a more rapid recovery.

Always evaluate:

1. Those tasks that the mastectomee, with your encouragement, can and should do for herself as part of her rehabilitation.

2. Those tasks that she should tackle only with a varying degree of help.

3. Those tasks that you would or should do for her even if she were 100 per cent fit.

12. 'Where Do I Go From Here?'

You must have noticed that at the main entrance to any clinic or hospital these days, you are immediately confronted by giant signboards directing you to 'Reception', 'Admissions', 'Out Patients Department', 'Physiotherapy', 'Pathology', 'X-ray', and so on. That is practical help on the way in. Wouldn't it be nice to find similar signs on the way out indicating just where you go for practical help once you are outside again?

Of course, it is not possible. We all have problems peculiar to ourselves and there would not be a signboard big enough to spell out all the answers.

'Where *do* I go from here?' 'Where do I begin?' 'Who's got the answer?' 'What's more – who wants the question?'

As you come out into the open again, you cannot help but feel that little bit 'alone'. And it is only as you leave hospital that you remember all those questions you forgot to ask!

No one is completely self-sufficient which is why in today's society people have learned to group together for mutual self-help.

The Mastectomy Association

But voluntary organizations do not just 'happen'. In every case, there must be a founder who can lead and organize and inspire and persuade others to get involved. The founder of the Mastectomy Association of Great Britain is Betty Westgate:

> You and I are not alone; many thousands of women have had a mastectomy, and for as far ahead as we can see, thousands more will have to undergo this operation. Without doubt it is one that causes anxiety and emotional distress.

I founded the Mastectomy Association in December 1973, simply in response to needs (expressed by women who had undergone a mastectomy) for an organization which could cater for their post-mastectomy needs. The main aim is to help women who have recently had, or been advised to have, a breast removed.

The services provided by members of the Association are strictly non-medical but designed to complement medical and nursing care. We can give practical information about bras, different types of prostheses and swimwear. We can also offer empathic understanding and support. At present, it seems that the woman who has herself experienced a mastectomy, and coped with the various problems it poses, can best offer this person-to-person advice.

The Association's activities are based on volunteer helpers throughout the country – each of whom has had the operation. To date, I have compiled a register of over 1000 volunteers whose names are listed in county registers and subdivided by age and family composition. This means that when a new 'client' asks for help, the volunteer most conveniently situated and most closely matching her for family experience can readily be put in touch with her by telephone, letter or visit.

In this way, a client may talk freely and without a time limit to someone with whom she shares a common experience, someone who has resumed her normal everyday life. This helps the 'client' to come to terms with the various aspects of her operation. Approximately 2500 women have applied for help of one sort or another. The Association publishes leaflets for the guidance of volunteer helpers and 'clients'.

The term 'client' is perhaps misleading, for the service is provided entirely free of charge. A number of members of the medical and nursing professions and social workers have sought information about the Association and are passing this on to their patients. Close co-operation with hospital and social workers will enable many women who need help to become aware of the Association; thousands of women will learn of its existence through this book. So often a patient is buoyed up by the staff and social activities of the ward; it is when she gets home and has to face the practical problems resulting from her mastectomy that she is apt to feel a little lonely and apprehensive and in need of help.

If you are interested in the Association or if you know of anyone who might benefit from contact, the address to write to is: Betty Westgate, The Mastectomy Association, 1 Colworth Road, Croydon CR0 7AD. (Telephone: 01-654 8643).

If you do decide to write, a stamped, addressed envelope would be appreciated.

Social Workers

Help of one kind or another is available from other sources, too. Betty mentioned that social workers have sought information on the mastectomy subject and are passing this on to their patients. This branch of the paramedical professions can be of assistance in many ways, yet there is a widespread belief that the only function of social workers is to sort out patient's financial problems.

Any stigma attached to being visited by a social worker is as unjustified as it would be to say that a nurse's only function is to empty bed-pans. It is true that social workers help the destitute, the down-and-outs, the alcoholics; but it is equally true that they are trained to *listen* and to give advice on a wide range of personal and family problems in addition to financial ones. Though there is a shortage of social workers in some areas, every major hospital has at least one experienced 'counsellor' on its staff.

Outside hospital, contact can be made through your local authority or you could phone or write to one of the voluntary social or welfare organizations. Each of these bodies (listed in the yellow pages of your phone book under Social Service and Welfare Organizations) has someone trained and willing to help with any community problem. You may find that some unexpected little trauma crops up long after you leave hospital. Do not let it become a mountain when there are social workers and mastectomy volunteers who could help you.

Fitting Salons

From a practical point of view, two manufacturers have

established salons where trained consultants demonstrate and fit comprehensive ranges of breastforms and mastectomy apparel. These are: The Mastectomy Centre, 12 Henrietta Place, London W1. (Telephone: 01-580 8575); Patientcare Ltd, Room 213, Bond Street House, 14 Clifford Street, London W1X 1RE. (Telephone: 01-491 4118).

Replacement Surgery

Should you be considering a breast implant under the National Health Scheme, you can either mention this when you go for your check-up at the hospital, or make an appointment to revisit your surgeon. If you have moved to another area, make an appointment to see a surgeon at your local hospital. Each case must be considered on its own merits before the patient can be referred to a plastic surgeon for a final decision about the possibility of surgery.

If you wish to have the surgery carried out privately, you should see your own doctor. Your doctor may then write to a plastic surgeon, and should the surgeon feel that he can help, he will arrange to see you prior to making a final decision. The current price for internal prostheses is in the order of £90 each; this is not inclusive of the surgeon's fee or any other expenses.

However, we feel that we should prepare you for the fact that not all medical people are enthusiastic about replacement surgery and there are those who hold strong convictions to the contrary, believing that it could hide further developments of cancer. Finally, not every mastectomee is suited either physically or by temperament.

Overcoming Depression

As we near the end of this book, there are still some issues we have not discussed. Some, such as whether or not you should have any more children and whether or not you should breast feed, must be left for your doctor's advice because each case (as with the question of implant surgery) is different. Other topics, such as the particular problems of unmarried mastectomees and lonely immigrants, are best left for you to discuss with a social worker or with a contact from a voluntary group.

Depression can be a self-perpetuating problem if you fail to realize that most mastectomees have periods of depression for varying periods after surgery and/or radiotherapy. Have some form of depression-antidote routine you can fall back on; a hairdo, a new dress, a funny record, a good book. To each her own, but do not get depressed because you are depressed!

Catapult yourself back to health by paying particular attention to a well-balanced diet. Avoid trashy foods. Buy or borrow a dietetic book or reputable health magazine to give you incentive and ideas. A new interest in a health-conscious diet can be a wonderful way of countering a tendency towards depression. There are now several hundred health food stores selling a wide variety of natural foodstuffs which are far more interesting and nutritious than our average diet of 'wheatybangs' and 'plastic' white bread. A Directory of Health Food Stores appears in *Here's Health* magazine, and although we do not necessarily subscribe to the claims of all the magazine's advertisers, the editorial matter contains a great deal of dietetic and nutritional sense. Suffice to say we welcome the trend away from synthetic additives and we guess you know how to be selective in regard to advertising matter anyway.

Just as we feel sure you will be sensible about any unhappy mastectomy reports you may read in the Press, remember that Betty, Janet, Kate, Ruth, Jean, Elizabeth, Ann and Vera are truly representative of the many thousands who have made complete recoveries. Indeed, it saddens us that we do not have space to share with you all the heartwarming stories that we have collected over the last two to three years.

Help From the Media

One last story illustrates the power of the communications media to do the maximum amount of good. Jessie is a 50-year-old bilateral mastectomee from Ilford, Essex:

One morning, nine months after an operation for a bilateral

mastectomy and having resumed most of my former activities, I found myself ironing away at the family wash with more than my usual vigour. The 'iron-bashing' was a symptom of my annoyance with a London hospital where, to my disgust, I had just been refused the National Health issue of the prosthesis that I felt was the one most suitable for me. In actual fact, the prosthesis I wanted was less expensive than the one the hospital had forced on me. The whole bureaucratic, nonsensical attitude of a low-level, male administrator incapable of understanding a simple feminine request, which would save the taxpayer money into the bargain, absolutely infuriated me.

Suddenly, I realized that the background voice on my radio was that of Katie Boyle whose forthright views on the mastectomy subject had been widely quoted in the Press. I must have been really angry or I just wouldn't have had the courage to do what I did next which was simply to bang down the iron, telephone the BBC and register my protest about the inadequacies of that particular hospital administrator!

Well, I got a sympathetic hearing all right but after I had erupted my annoyance all over the network, I sat back and trembled and wondered if I had done the right thing.

Two hours later, I was safely convinced that I had when a personal telephone call from Katie Boyle (something I hadn't dreamed of!) came through, in which she told me that she had arranged for me to visit a privately run centre in London. I also had a confirmatory telephone call from the manufacturers concerned. Just one week later I had a brand new 'you can't tell the difference' bustline and a chance meeting with Ian Swash.

I sincerely hope that the book is a success, as I feel it will be beneficial to so many women. I wish that I had experienced the companionship, support and practical help of it during my hospitalization and in the early stages of rehabilitation when I often felt unique in my problem.

At least I could have waved the relevant sections of it under the nose of that chauvinist male. Perhaps someone could see that he gets a copy! Meanwhile, I continue to go from strength to strength. My mastectomy is no longer an affliction and my next step is to learn to drive in the hope that, once completely mobile, I shall be able to play a part in the rehabilitation of other mastectomees.

Things have gone well for me since my impromptu broadcast.

The day that I was told I had cancer of the breast was a dismal one, but I am stronger for the experience and every single day since then has been brighter than the days that went before.

I can congratulate myself on being a very happy woman; fit and well and so very much alive.

Jessie's heartwarming story brings us full circle at the point where she, in her turn, sets out to help others.

As we close this chat with you, our hope is that no matter what your background or environment or personality, you will strive to make the same good recovery; and that the blessings of your life will be intensified.

A friend said: 'I pledged myself to begin that day with hope for tomorrow, and each tomorrow with a little more hope for the next and so on. It just struck me the other day, that over the last fifteen years or so, it seems to have worked pretty well.'

Glossary of Terms

Benign: When speaking of a tumour or growth or lump, benign means *not* malignant, i.e. *not* cancerous.

Bilateral: In respect of mastectomy, the removal of *both* breasts.

Biopsy: The removal of tissue for microscopic examination.

Carcinoma: Medical term for cancerous growth.

Cervix: Neck of womb.

Implant: The surgical insertion of an internal prosthesis.

Lumpectomy: The removal of a malignant lump without the removal of a breast.

Malignant: Cancerous.

Oopherectomy: Surgical removal of the ovaries.

Prognosis: The medical prediction of a patient's future.

Prosthesis: A replacement for any part of the body, so a mammary prosthesis is a false breast or breastform. Derived from words meaning 'an addition'.

Radiotherapy: Treatment by radiation.

Manufacturers and Associations

Main Manufacturers and Distributors of Mastectomy Apparel

Great Britain
S.H. Camp & Company Limited, East Portway, Andover, Hants SP10 3NL. (Telephone: 0264 63173)

Ross & Hilliard (Patientcare), 33 Albert Square, Dundee DD1 1DJ. (Telephone: 0382 21593)

Spencer (Banbury) Limited, Britannia Road, Banbury, Oxon. (Telephone: 0295 2265)

The Medical Supply Association: Bourne Road, Bexley, Kent DA5 1LF. (Telephone: Crayford 29114)

Strodex House, Nottingham Road, Long Eaton, Notts. (Telephone: Long Eaton 2203)

Torplay, Torpoint, St Bees, Whitehaven, Cumbria. (Telephone: 094 685 225 and 0946 5157)

Southern Ireland
P.E.I. Limited, 13 Fade Street, Dublin 2. (Telephone: Dublin 770142)

U.S.A.
Airway Surgical Company, Erie Avenue, Cincinnati, Ohio 45209. Telephone: (513) 271-4594

ATCO Surgical Supports Co., 450 Portage Trail/Cuyahoga Falls, Ohio 44222. Telephone: (216) 928-2153

Berger Brothers Company, Confidante Division, 135 Derby Avenue, New Haven, Conn. 06507. Telephone: (203) 624-0131

Camp International, Jackson, Mich.

Identical Form, Inc., 17 W. 60th Street, New York, N.Y. 10023. Telephone: (212) 586-3708

Jodee Bra, Inc., 200 Madison Avenue, New York. Telephone: (212) 689-3005

Miriam Gates (Helene Barrie, Inc.), 289 Skidmore Road, Deer Park, N.Y. Telephone: (516) 242-2262

Stryker Corporation, 420 Alcott Street, Kalamazoo, Michigan 49001. Telephone: (616) 381-3811

Mail Order

Sears, Roebuck and Co., North Philadelphia Station, Philadelphia, Pa.19132

Australia

Bosclip Distributors, 45 Meeks Road, Marrickville 2204.

Downs Surgical (Aust) Pty Ltd, 575 George Street, Sydney 2000.

Femmeline, 105 Main Street, Croydon 3136.

Jenyns Corset Pty Ltd, 223 Albert Street, Brisbane 4000.

V. Mayes & Co, 903 Nepean Highway, Moorabbin 3189.

Muir & Neil Pty Ltd, 497 Kent Street, Sydney 2000.

Nursu Wools, 230 Main North Road, Prospect 5082.

Main Manufacturers and Distributors of Lymphoedema Appliances

Great Britain

Flowtron-Aire Limited, 5A Lye Trading Estate, 137-141 Old Bedford Road, Luton, Beds LU2 4BR. (Telephone: 0582 413104/5/6)

Ross & Hilliard, 33 Albert Square, Dundee DD1 1DJ. (Telephone: 0382 21593)

Australia
See Surgical Appliances in yellow pages, or Buyers' Guide of telephone directories.

Manufacturers and Distributors of Arm Sleeves
E. Sallis Ltd., Vernon Works, Basford, Nottingham, NG6 0DH. (Telephone: Nottingham 77841-2 and 75452)

Department Stores Stocking a Wide Range of Mastectomy Apparel
D.H. Evans, 318 Oxford Street, London W1.
Clements (Watford), 29 The Parade, High Street, Watford, Herts.

Mastectomy Associations
The Mastectomy Association of Great Britain, 1 Colworth Road, Croydon CR0 7AD. (Telephone: 01-654 8643)

The Mastectomy Association of Southern Ireland, 14 Effra Road, Dublin 6.

Mastectomy Advisory Programme of The Ulster Cancer Foundation, 40 Eglantine Avenue, Belfast BT9 6DX. (Telephone: Belfast 663281/2).

(See also under Educational/Voluntary Services).

Mastectomy Fitting Centres
The Mastectomy Centre, 12 Henrietta Place, London W1. (Telephone: 01-580 8575)

Australia: Most city and provincial department stores and some boutiques – see lists prepared by Australian Cancer Society, Sydney.

Patientcare
(Centres providing a comprehensive range of mastectomy apparel, lymphoedema pumps and elastic sleeves)

Room 213, Bond Street House, 14 Clifford Street, London W1X 1RE. (Telephone: 01-491 4118)

22 Union Street, Dundee DD1 4BH. (Telephone: 0382 26161)

121 Douglas Street, Glasgow G2 4HE. (Telephone: 041-332 4414)

37-39 George IV Bridge, Edinburgh EH1 1EL. (Telephone: 031-226 5125)

8-10 Union Street, Inverness. (Telephone: 0463 36691)

For details of new centres and/or home fitting services throughout the UK, write to Patientcare Mastectomy Centres, 33 Albert Square, Dundee DD1 1DJ.

In Australia, contact the Breast Clinic or Senior Social Worker of nearest Public Hospital.

Medic Alert Foundation

Medic Alert Foundation, 9 Hanover Street, London W1. (Telephone: 01-499 2261)

In the USA: Medic-Alert, 1000 N. Palm Street, PO Box 1009, Purlock, California.

In Australia: Medic-Alert, 21a Austin Street, Adelaide 5000. (Telephone: 08/223 1316).

Cancer Information Services (including breast screening)

Cancer Information Association, Marigold House, Carfax, Oxford OX1 1EF. (Telephone: 0865 46654 or 0865 725223).

The Medical Centre, BUPA, Webb House, 210 Pentonville Road, Kings Cross, London N1 9TA. (Telephone: 01-278 4565/4647)

Australian Cancer Society, Cnr King and Castlereagh Streets, Sydney 2000. (Telephone: 02/231 3355).

Camperdown Diagnostic Centre, Suite 117, 9 Missenden Road, Camperdown 2050. (Telephone: 02/516 3266). (Provides a comprehensive screening service for women from any area of Australia).

Educational/Voluntary Services

International Association of Cancer Victims and Friends (IACVF), PO Box 3718, Beverley Hills, Ca 90212.

In Australia: Mastectomy Rehabilitation Service, c/o Australian Cancer Society, Cnr King and Castlereagh Streets, Sydney 2000. (Telephone: 02/231 3355).

Reading List

If you have an enquiring mind, the following books could be of interest to you as supplementary reading. The list is offered only as a broad outline of the possibilities; if these titles are not available, consult your librarian or bookseller for substitutes.

Atoms At Tea Time, Pia Paoli. (Andre Deutsch, London.)
The story of a cure.
Cancer and Commonsense, George Crile Jnr, MD. (Robert Hale, London.)
What Women Should Know About the Breast Cancer Controversy, George Crile Jnr, MD. (Pocket Books, New York.)
Determined to Live, Brian Hession. (Peter Davies, London.)
A book that has brought comfort, courage and inspiration to many people in many countries.
Dressmaking Made Simple, Gidon Lippman ASIA and Dorothy Erskins. (W.H. Allen, London.)
My Friend Says It's Bulletproof, Penelope Mortimer. (Hutchinson, London.)
A mastectomee proves to herself, in the oldest way known to womankind, that she is still feminine. Light fiction.
Overcoming Depression, Paul Hauck. (Sheldon Press, London.)
Reach to Recovery, Terese Lasser and William Kendall Clarke. (Simon & Schuster, New York.)
The story of one woman's victory over the emotional and physical impact of breast surgery.
Relax, Jane Madders, illustrated by Richard Bonson. (BBC Publications, London.)

'My Doctor kept telling me to relax and I knew he was right but I simply didn't know how.' This book teaches you.

The Nature of Cancer, P.M. Sutton, BSc, MB, BS, MCPath. (The English Universities Press, London.)

The Complete Book of Handicrafts (Sewing, Knitting, Crochet, Dyecraft, Spinning and Weaving, Embroidery, Macramé, Tapestry, Leathercraft, Rugmaking) (Hamlyn, exclusively for W.H. Smith.)

For beginners onwards. Each skill is compartmentalized in its own section for easy reference. 'A springboard to creativity.'

The Climate is Hope by Walter Ross. (First published by Prentice Hall Inc., thereafter by Lansdowne Press, and distributed in Great Britain by George Newnes Limited, London.)

'This book helps to eliminate unwarranted fear of cancer. It shows that early detection and medical advances make cancer one of the most curable of all major diseases' – Leonard W. Larson, past President, The American Medical Association.

Afterword

In the last decade, numerous books and articles have been written about cancer in general. They fall broadly into three categories; those written by the medical profession, those written by investigative journalists, and those written by the patient.

All are valuable, but often do not fulfil the requirements of the lay person, either being too non-specific or too medically incomprehensible. And although breast cancer is four times as common as cervical cancer, for example, nowhere, until now, has the mastectomy patient been able to find a practical guide to rehabilitation.

I commend this book to new patients as the first of its kind to be published in Britain. I recommend it as compulsive reading to fellow members of the medical and paramedical professions who rightly see the patient as the central figure in the medical team; and to all those who value the quality of human life.

There are few homes today which have not known something of the ravages of cancer and the anxiety and fear that it occasions. I am pleased to note the importance that the authors place on early diagnosis and the routine of self-examination, for early treatment means a much higher cure-rate. It is hoped that the use of case histories will enable women to identify with those who have faced their mastectomies with courage and equanimity so that they, in turn, may become equally inspired. The case histories also indicate that breast cancer is a slow growing disease, so slow that many women fail to discern any increase in the tumour, even over a period of weeks. A woman who finds a lump in her breast should not wait to see if it gets larger or simply hope that it will go away; she should consult her family doctor *immediately*.

In all, this is a warm, very human and immensely practical book and one that has a special part to play in the lives of many thousands of women and their families.

GILBERT H. COLLIER, CStJ, MRCS, LRCP, MRCGP, FRSM

Index